COPING TOGETHER, SIDE BY SIDE

Enriching Mother-Daughter Communication Across the Breast Cancer Journey

HEALTH COMMUNICATION

Gary L. Kreps, *series editor*

Handbook of Patient-Provider Interactions: Raising and Responding to Concerns About Life, Illness, and Disease
Wayne Beach (ed.)

A Natural History of Family Cancer
Wayne Beach

Death: The Beginning of a Relationship
Christine S. Davis

Dirty Tale: A Narrative Journey of the IBD Body
Nichole L. Defenbaugh

Rhetoric of Healthcare: Essays Toward a New Disciplinary Inquiry
Barbara Heifferon & *Stuart C. Brown (eds.)*

Changing the Culture of College Drinking: A Socially Situated Health Communication Campaign
Linda C. Lederman & *Lea P. Stewart*

Health Communication and Faith Communities
Ann Neville Miller and Donald Rubin (eds.)

Handbook of Communication and Cancer Care
Dan O'Hair, Gary L. Kreps, & *Lisa Sparks, (eds.)*

Building the Evidence Base in Cancer Communication
Lila J. Finney Rutten, Bradford W. Hesse, Richard P. Moser, and Gary L. Kreps (eds.)

Crisis Communication and the Public Health
Matthew Seeger & *Timothy Sellnow (eds.)*

Cancer, Communication and Aging
Lisa Sparks, Dan O'Hair, & *Gary L. Kreps (eds.)*

Cancer and Death: A Love Story in Two Voices
Leah Vande Berg and Nick Trujillo

Communicating About HIV/AIDS: Taboo Topics and Difficult Conversations
Kandi L. Walker, Joy L. Hart, and Margaret D'Silva (eds.)

E-Health: The Advent of Online Cancer Information Systems
Pamela Whitten, Gary L. Kreps, and Matthew S. Eastin

Communicating Spirituality in Health Care
Maggie Wills (ed.)

COPING TOGETHER, SIDE BY SIDE

Enriching Mother-Daughter Communication Across the Breast Cancer Journey

Carla L. Fisher, Ph.D.

George Mason University

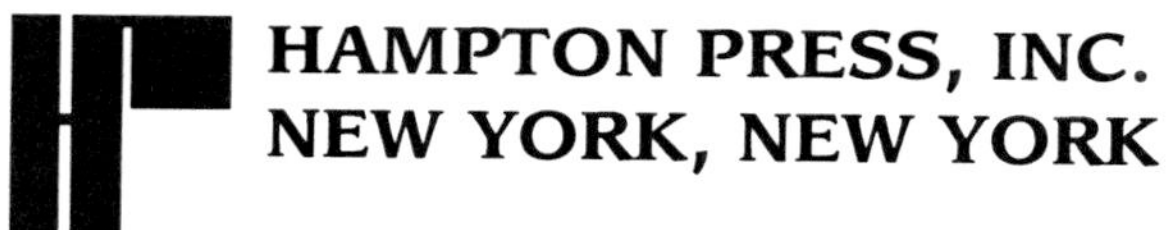

HAMPTON PRESS, INC.
NEW YORK, NEW YORK

Printed in the United States of America

Library of Congress Cataloging-in-Publication Data

Fisher, Carla L., author
Coping together, side by side : enriching mother-daughter communication across the breast cancer journey / Carla L. Fisher
p. ; cm. -- (Health communication)
Includes bibliographical references and indexes
ISBN 978-1-61289-140-8 (hardbound) -- ISBN 978-1-61289-141-5 (paperbound)
I. Title. II. Series: Health communication (New York, N.Y.)
[DNLM: 1. Breast neoplasms--psychology. 2. Adaptation, Psychological, 3. Interpersonal relations. 4. Parent-Child Relations. WP 870]
RC280.B8
616.99'449--dc23

201409666

Hampton Press, Inc.
307 Seventh Avenue
New York, NY 10001

She was by my side.
My mother was by my side. . . .
She took a very big part of being my partner. . . .
She set the standard for everyone else.
~A diagnosed daughter

Her pain was my pain. . . .
I feel like if she's with me, then
everything is okay because I know she's okay.
~Mother of a diagnosed daughter

~ ~ ~ ~ ~ ~ ~ ~ ~ ~ ~ ~ ~ ~ ~~ ~ ~~ ~ ~ ~ ~ ~~

It's just that she's there and she's concerned,
and she's there no matter what.
~A diagnosed mother

My mom says,
"I didn't go through this. We did."
It's like our thing.
~Daughter of a diagnosed mother

In loving memory of
My aunt Rosemary Lois (Paule) Oldendorph
and her mother, my grandmother,
Lucretia Genevieve (Bross) Paule

In honor of
Rose's daughters (Diane, Yvonne, Carla, & Laura)
Rose's granddaughters (Carrie, Melissa, Tara, Stephanie,
Nichole, Michelle, & Brittany)
Rose's great-granddaughters (Tayler, Olivia, Onalee, Rylan,
Mati, Kristin, Ashleigh, Emma, Katy, & Jordyn)
Rose's sisters (Patricia, Carleen, Barbara, Kathryn, & Deborah)
My mother, Deborah Ann (Paule) Fisher
All of the mothers and daughters who graciously
shared their stories with me

Dedicated to
My daughter,
Isa Luciana Fisher Muñoz
You are all that my heart ever desired

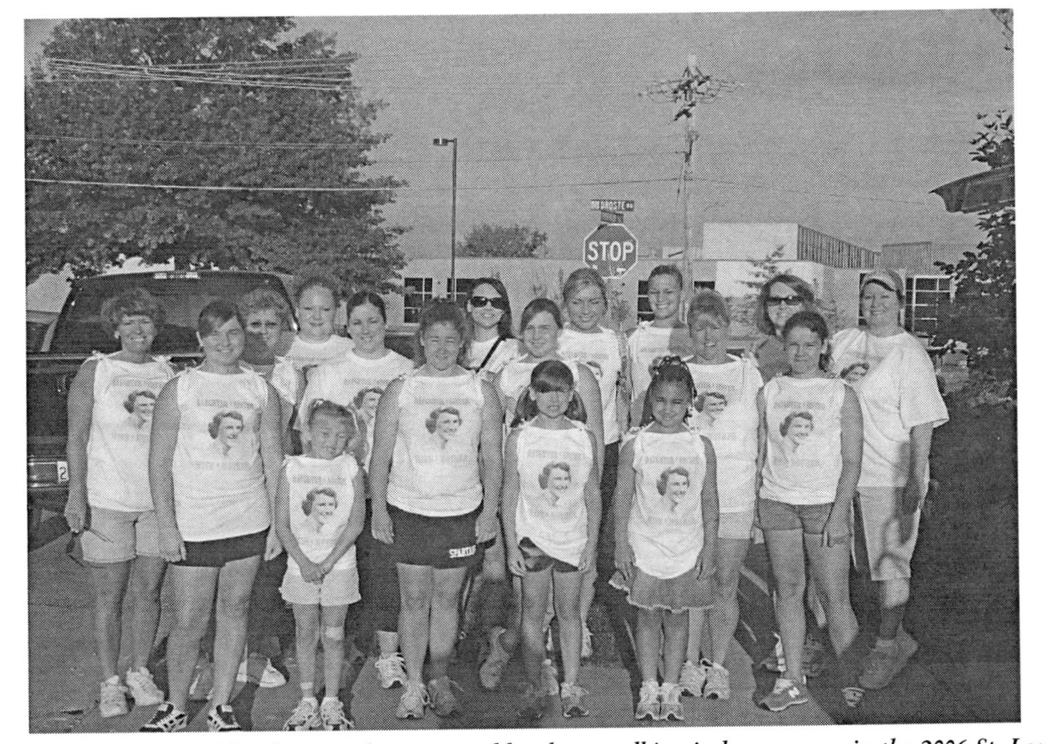

Rose's daughters, granddaughters, and great-granddaughters walking in her memory in the 2006 St. Louis Race for the Cure . Photo: Dan Foust.

CONTENTS

Part IV
The Centrality of Family Communication to Wellness After a Cancer Diagnosis

Part V
Secrecy and Sharing Among Mothers and Daughters: Exploring Openness and Avoidance

Part VI
Coping Side by Side: Adaptive and Maladaptive Emotional Support

Part VII
Journaling Mother-Daughter Communication During Treatment: Triangulating Findings

Part VIII
Enhancing Mothers' and Daughters' "Psychosocial Map" of Breast Cancer

FOREWORD

Two magnificent waves have been sweeping over the community of behavioral scientists who investigate the internal and external lives of humans. The first wave centers on the new technologies that enable us to view the physical dynamics of the brain/body. We can see and better understand the processes of cognition and emotion. Each day we become more aware of the interconnectivity of the brain and have concluded that our brains are so big (compared with other social mammals, bees, ants, etc.) and use so much of our caloric input because of our complex social/relational world. We need the big brain and so much energy to help us manage our social interactions. The second wave moves those of us who study human behavior and interaction to better communicate our theories and research findings to a much larger lay audience. We need to "translate" the fundamental knowledge advances of our work as well as actively participate within the interventions that significantly improve the lives of each and every person who shares our world.

The trap that a great many behavioral scientists fall into as we become caught up within the scientific surf of these waves is to focus solely on the activity within the brain/body. We become obsessed with the colorful pictures of brain activity or the interconnectivity within the brain as we compare healthy, "normal" brains with unhealthy "abnormalities." We seem to forget that the brain is a social tool. The most advanced technologies that map brain activity are only the first, most reductionistic step in our understanding of how humans behave and interact with one another in a complex relational world. The working memory and mentalizing functions of the brain/body that neuroscientists Matthew Lieberman (2013) and Joshua

Greene (2013) have so competently translated into readable texts ignore the actual process of socializing, of supporting, of relationship maintenance and change.

Carla Fisher has written a book that moves us significantly beyond the first wave and the "brain/body trap" by moving outside of an individual brain/body to focus on the dynamic, communicative nature of the mother-daughter relationship following a diagnosis of breast cancer. She accomplishes the goal of the second wave by writing a book written for a wide audience of family members, friends, and healthcare providers. In essence, this book focuses our attention on a third wave of scientific discovery: to describe and understand how our communication constructs a breast cancer diagnosis as fundamentally relational.

Coping Together, Side by Side: Enriching Mother-Daughter Communication Across the Breast Cancer Journey focuses on our communication within the mother-daughter relationship as they co-manage a diagnosis of breast cancer. Carla views breast cancer as much more than a cellular destroying process. Breast cancer is more than an internal dynamic of brain and body. A diagnosis of breast cancer is fundamentally relational. Managing breast cancer is a mother-daughter relational journey. This relational journey impacts how this disease is understood, how this disease is successfully managed and possibly destroyed, and how the physical, emotional, and relational components of the mother-daughter relationship move forward to impact the quality of life for both mothers and daughters. Carla identifies the complex interactive dynamics of this intergenerational relationship. Carla uses the words of mothers and daughters to shed light on the breast cancer experience. She then links a greater understanding of the mother-daughter relationship to possible improved interventions that aid both healthcare workers and other family members and friends to accomplish successful interventions.

Carla Fisher has written a landmark book that greatly expands our understanding of breast cancer. She expertly underscores the impactful and fundamental relational nature of a breast cancer diagnosis. She enriches our understanding of the mother-daughter relationship as a fluid, dynamic, and essential component of the breast cancer experience. Carla, then, links her research findings to pragmatic interventions to aid all of us as we, or our loved ones, cope with a diagnosis of breast cancer. She leaves us with insight, hope, and a new vision for understanding the fundamental relational nature of not only breast cancer but all challenges that life offers.

Jon F. Nussbaum, PhD
Professor of Communication Arts & Sciences
and Human Development & Family Studies
The Pennsylvania State University

ACKNOWLEDGMENTS

This research and book would not exist were it not for the generosity, patience, guidance, and kindness of many wonderful people. First and foremost, I would like to thank all of the women who have participated in my research. Thank you for welcoming me into your lives. I am grateful to all of you for honoring me with your candid stories of unified strength, courage, and resilience. Thank you also to Dr. Gary Kreps, who has tirelessly supported my research and this book and been a most wonderful colleague, and to Barbara Bernstein and Hampton Press for your faith, support, and patience. I am also immensely grateful to Heather Jefferson for her incredibly keen copyediting eye and instrumental insight.

A special thanks to Drs. Jon Nussbaum, Michelle Miller-Day, Dennis Gouran, and Melissa Hardy for your influential support and guidance on the foundational study. I am also eternally grateful for having had such incredible mentors across my graduate training and during my research career (Drs. Jon Nussbaum, Michelle Miller-Day, Vincent Waldron, Jeffrey Kassing, Doug Kelley, Carma Bylund, Dennis Gouran, Kory Floyd, Steve Zarit, Melissa Hardy, and Don Boileau). I admire each of you as a researcher and teacher but also as a friend. Each of you has been exceedingly giving of your time, wisdom, and encouragement. Thank you for teaching me the art and science of meaningful interdisciplinary research.

I am especially thankful to two mentors in particular who are like family to me, and, without them, this foundational study would never have been possible. I will always be so grateful to have had Dr. Jon F. Nussbaum as my doctoral advisor and NIA preceptor. You have always given me just the right amount of guidance and independence to allow me to pave my own path as a scholar. Your work and humanity will continuously inspire me, and I am so grateful to have your lifelong mentorship and friendship. I am also immensely indebted to Dr. Michelle A. Miller-Day. Your enthusiasm, wisdom, and honesty have been endless and selfless. Thank you for helping me "learn to see" as a researcher and for being such a fun, loving friend. You both set the standard for being the best mentors and friends.

Thank you to all of the individuals and organizations who helped me recruit women to participate in the foundational study. A special thanks to Aileen S. Galley, ACSW, LSW, Kristin Sides, BS, and the research board of Mount Nittany Medical Center and Mount Nittany Physician Group (formerly Centre Medical and Surgical Associates); Hershey Medical Center and the Women's Health Center and Breast Imaging, particularly Susann E. Schetter, DO, Anne Bobb, BSN, RN, CWOCN, and Shanna K. Gillette, BS, RTR(M); and the Kathryn Candor Lundy Breast Health Center, especially Diane Sholder, RN, BSN, OCN. Thank you to Lillie Shockney, RN, BS, MAS, Charmayne Dierker, and the board of Mothers Supporting Daughters with Breast Cancer (MSDBC) for taking the time to talk with me about your experiences. A special thanks as well to Mayo Clinic of Arizona (especially Dean Teresa Britt Pipe, PhD, RN) and Memorial Sloan-Kettering Cancer Center's Department of Psychiatry and Behavioral Sciences (especially Carma Bylund, PhD) for engaging in related ongoing collaborative research with me.

I was also fortunate to receive funding from the following institutions to conduct this research and complete the book: the National Institute on Aging (NIA Training Grant: T32 AG00048) and The Pennsylvania State University's Gerontology Center; the Joseph M. Juran Center for Leadership in Quality; Penn State's College of the Liberal Arts; Arizona State University's New College; and George Mason University. Thank you also to the following colleagues and research assistants for their collaboration or assistance on data analyses, presentation of findings, and construction of this book with both the foundational study data and related extensions of this study: Dr. Craig Fowler, Dr. Bianca Wolf, Nicole Piemonte, Mollie Rose Canzona, and Emily Peterson.

I am very grateful to my friends and family for their continuous support of my research and finishing this book. A special thanks to my parents (Lynn and Debbie) who taught me early on the importance of family interaction and sharing stories, my brothers (Carson and Collin) for always being there for me and making many memorable stories with me, and four treasured friends (Brandi Gancarz, Nicole Leicht, Khadi Ndiaye, and Bianca Wolf) for keeping it real with their immense kindness, enthusiasm, comic relief, unwavering support, and sisterhood. Finally, I am very grateful for the love and encouragement of my husband, Christopher Muñoz, and our daughter, Isa Luciana Fisher Muñoz. Chris, you uphold integrity and compassion in every aspect of your being, and your beautiful soul inspires me every day. Isa Lu, your smiles, laughter, and sweet happy spirit make us whole. Thank you for playing gleefully (and patiently) while I wrote feverishly. Every smile, babble, and giggle helped me pull through. I am so thankful to have a life with you all.

INTRODUCTION

The interpersonal communication that fuels our social world is as essential to our survival as any biological or physical process that keeps us alive.
(Hummert, Nussbaum, & Wiemann, 1994, p. 3)

Communication is a fundamental part of being—the core of family. It builds kin relationships, maintains family networks, and enables individuals to achieve life satisfaction. Although rarely prioritized in society, communication is one key to a high quality of life.

Family communication is especially important when we encounter traumatic changes that disrupt everyday life. Stress and coping research indicates that "the way people cope is largely a function of their interaction with others" (Afifi & Nussbaum, 2006, p. 282). What we must also better recognize is that our family interactions can function both adaptively and maladaptively (be helpful or unhelpful) when we adjust to strenuous circumstances. In other words, we do not always communicate with one another in a healthy manner, even when we think we are being supportive.

Rather, we are human. We are not born with innate communication aptitude for any situation—communication competence is something we gain across the life span as we expand our social experiences (Pecchioni, Wright, & Nussbaum, 2005). When families encounter stressful transitions, such as life-threatening diagnoses, they need to incorporate new strategies or behavioral approaches to adapt effectively (Cowan, 1991). Given this, it is important for behavioral scientists to investigate family communication during health crises so that we can better assist them in learning to interact in ways that enhance their ability to adapt and emerge resilient across the life span.

In our modern-day world, the diagnosis and treatment of cancer is a stressful transition that families frequently encounter. In our society, the word *cancer* brings with it a multitude of distressing assumptions. As the second leading cause of death in the United States (Hoyert, Kung, & Smith, 2005), a diagnosis of cancer might be one of the most difficult challenges a family will face across the life span. How families communicate during such crises plays a role in their ability to emerge resilient (Walsh, 1996, 2006).

Psychosocial research shows that a patient's family interactions are critical to his or her well-being and adjustment to the disease (Goldsmith, Miller, & Caughlin, 2008; Hagedoorn et al., 2000; Pistrang, Barker, & Rutter, 1997). However, it is important to note that much of the research is focused on marital partners. While patients certainly rely on their spouse for support, the prioritization of this relationship in research negates the reality that for patients diagnosed with certain types of cancer, *other* family bonds may be especially important to their coping. This might be particularly true for women facing breast cancer. The mother-daughter relationship has emerged in a select few studies as an important factor in women's adjustment to breast cancer (Burles, 2006; Oktay & Walter, 1991; Spira & Kenemore, 2000).

Breast cancer afflicts more than 200,000 women each year, adding to more than 2 million women already living with the disease (Jemel et al., 2003). According to the National Cancer Institute (NCI), a component of the National Institutes of Health (NIH), 1 in 8 women born today will develop breast cancer during their lifetime. The World Health Organization (WHO) estimates that nearly a half million women will lose their life to the disease each year. Across the globe, this reality is not overlooked. We have an entire month dedicated to fighting this disease as a society. The majority of our population likely has some awareness of what it means to be afflicted with this disease. At the very least, we recognize what a pink ribbon refers to or why so many grocery products, such as soup cans, have pink labels in October.

Thanks in part to advocacy efforts like Susan G. Komen and the National Breast Cancer Coalition, the face of breast cancer in society has changed over the last few decades. A "pink ribbon culture" has emerged, bringing with it a social movement aimed at improving women's health care. Gone is the day when people would cross the street just to avoid someone they knew had cancer or when most families silenced each other from talking about it. The older women I talk to remember these days. The younger women often have no idea a day like that existed. Breast cancer is now a prominently discussed health issue, and advocacy efforts such as races for the cure make it a frequent presence in everyday life.

Less discussed in society, however, is how this disease ultimately afflicts not just the woman but her family, particularly her mother and/or daughter. For many women, breast cancer is a mother-daughter journey. For nearly a decade, the world heard about Elizabeth Edwards, wife of politician John Edwards, and her struggle with metastatic breast cancer. She became a national symbol of hope, strength, and tenacity as we all watched her family bind together to fight this disease, even in the midst of other family crises. Although the impact of her cancer experience on her daughters has rarely (if ever) been discussed, a year after her death, her adult daughter, Cate, wrote about how she supported her mother, often holding her hand (as her mother had always done for her) as she succumbed to the disease (2011). Cate Edwards described her profound connection to her mother even today, stating, "Mom feels so alive to me today. I think about her constantly. I hear her voice in every choice I make, big and small."

This book is an effort to further expand this social movement by better recognizing that breast cancer is a *shared mother-daughter experience*. Regardless of age at diagnosis, women have described their mother-daughter bond as an important part of their cancer-coping experience, both for the good and the bad, and this impact lasts well after treatment ends or a mother or daughter has died (Oktay & Walter, 1991). The significance of this kin bond for mothers and daughters encountering breast cancer is not entirely surprising given that the mother-daughter relationship is often the longest, most emotionally connected bond a woman will experience in her lifetime (Fischer, 1986). Yet this relationship is complicated—as is breast cancer—and mothers and daughters need help learning to communicatively navigate this disease and collectively fight it.

Unfortunately, most families will not have this need attended to in their oncology care. Too often health care addresses only patients' individually focused biomedical needs. When psychosocial treatment is available, patients often do not know about it given the lack of awareness in society about the role of family and psychology in cancer coping (Suinn, 1999). As a result, families enter the world of cancer without a "psychosocial map" to help guide their behavior as they attempt to adjust and cope with the disease together (Rolland, 1994; Rolland & Williams, 2005). Rather, family is often ignored in a patient's care regimen (Baider & Kaplan De-Noor, 2000).

The NCI's mission is in part to support research that can help families cope by eliminating suffering. Their mission addresses the "Cancer Control Continuum," which appreciates the entire disease trajectory or five aspects of cancer: prevention, detection, diagnosis, treatment, and survivorship. NCI identifies "communications" (which includes human communication or verbal and nonverbal behavior) as a significant issue influencing outcomes in each area (Kreuter, Green, Capella, Slater, & Clark, 2007). Yet psychosocial research on how families can cope with breast cancer in healthy ways is still lacking and certainly needed to enhance families' health promotion behavior, disease adjustment, resilience, and even survival.

This book serves to portray breast cancer as not just a family experience but a mother-daughter one. The tapestry of stories of the women presented herein invite families, clinicians, therapists, and researchers into this mother-daughter journey. These narratives represent both the difficulty and beauty mothers and daughters encounter after a diagnosis as they struggle to cope and support one another at various points in the life span. As a behavioral health scientist, I have surveyed and talked with hundreds of mothers and daughters one on one about their experiences. I began this research with one large foundational study in which I surveyed and talked to women diagnosed at different ages—in young adulthood, midlife, and later life—who selflessly shared with me their mother-daughter journey with this disease. This book presents the findings from this foundational study as well as extended studies encompassing my larger research program on mother-daughter breast cancer communication. I have conducted this research in an effort to both improve psycho-oncology care by capturing how family behavior impacts a diagnosed woman's ability to cope and heighten the importance of family communication to the medical community and society at large. At the same time, this research demonstrates the importance of mother-daughter communication in the context of breast cancer.

This book might be of use to health behavior researchers and students, practitioners, interventionists, as well as families who encounter breast cancer. The stories presented herein can provide a deeper understanding of the social side of cancer or family dynamics during illness and how that connects to our overall quality of life. As such, this book could serve as a resource across disciplines concerned with health, illness, and family behavior such as communication, aging and human development, family studies, therapy, nursing, public health, developmental psychology, and psycho-oncology. Given the mixed-method research design and triangulation of data, this book might also provide students and scientists with an example of ways to blend paradigms and mix data to get a fuller picture of health and behavior.

Ultimately, I hope my research expands health practitioners' perspectives of patients by bringing their voice to the forefront of the illness experience and simultaneously provides rich knowledge for intervention-making, thereby contributing to that "psychosocial map" of fighting cancer. At the same time, I hope that this book provides families with information that can ease their navigation of this disease course. Most important, I hope that mothers and daughters faced with this disease can find themselves in the stories of the women depicted in this book and, in doing so, better understand one another as they learn to communicate and connect while taking on breast cancer together.

Part I

MOTHERS, DAUGHTERS, AND BREAST CANCER

1

LINKED LIVES

The Story of Mothers and Daughters Across the Life Span

Linked lives ...
Tangled vines ...
Velvet chains ...
Lives together, worlds apart ...
Enduring bonds ...
A blood hyphen ...
Mirrored lives ...
Mixed emotions ...
Friends for life ...
The mother-daughter bond.[1]

To understand the mother-daughter legacy of breast cancer, one must begin with an appreciation of this profound linkage. The mother-daughter tie has been described in many different ways, some referencing selfless loyalty and love whereas others highlight friction and discord. The mother-daughter relationship can be both deeply intimate *and* tremendously complex.

[1]These references to the mother-daughter bond were extracted from a multitude of texts about maternal relationships from various scholarly perspectives.

Some mothers and daughters experience "linked lives" (Fischer, 1986)—an intimacy that binds them together as "velvet chains—chains of security, love, and devotion" (Miller-Day, 2004, p. 4). Mothers and daughters can be each other's crutch—their confidant and friend or advisor and nurturer. Yet even with an enduring connection that crosses generational boundaries, mothers and daughters might also feel "worlds apart" in the midst of complicated, "mixed emotions" (Fingerman, 2003; Walters, 1992). Their lives intertwine and tangle in unique ways that distinguish them from other relational ties, thereby complicating how they relate to one another. Many scholars and practitioners have argued that no other relationship in a woman's life can encounter such "blinding closeness, overwhelming joy, and intimidating anger" (Lifshin, 1992). In essence, the mother-daughter connection is a persistent, eternal vine—for some, a "blood hyphen" (Miller-Day, 2004, p. 4). Theirs is a colorful story of love and resilience.

A life-span, developmental perspective of the mother-daughter relationship allows one to tell the mother-daughter story across time—to encapsulate their relational history (Pecchioni, Wright, & Nussbaum, 2005). This framework emphasizes how mothers and daughters negotiate their connection at various points across the life span, which allows us to witness how critical their communication can be when adjusting to changes such as a breast cancer diagnosis.

UNDERSTANDING THE MOTHER-DAUGHTER CONNECTION ACROSS TIME: A DEVELOPMENTAL LENS

As journalist Victoria Secunda stated, "A daughter is a mother's gender partner, her closest ally in the family confederacy, an extension of herself. And mothers are their daughters' role model, their biological and emotional road map, the arbiter of all their relationships" (1992, p. 54). This profound connection (and at times divide) that mothers and daughters encounter across time has been widely studied in various disciplines as well as depicted in popular culture.

Some illustrations, such as well-known author Nancy Friday's (1977) renowned text *My Mother/My Self*, explore the powerful influence this bond has on a woman's psychological development. Friday explored the impact of a mother on her daughter's emotions, identity, sexuality, and self-esteem across the entirety of her life. Others, such as Secunda's (1991) *When You and Your Mother Can't Be Friends*, writer and pastoral counselor Kim Chernin's (1999) *The Woman Who Gave Birth to Her Mother*, and therapist Dr. Karyl McBride's (2008) *Will I Ever Be Good Enough?* all serve to help women heal from a difficult "mother story" or past. Their works provide women an opportunity to both open the future and break a pattern of hurtful mother-daughter behavior. Mother-daughter portrayals in movies and television are also widespread, with most dramatizing conflicting feelings of love and hate. These media depictions are important given that they influence how mothers and daughters evaluate their own relationships (O'Briend, 2011; Walters, 1992). At times popular culture offers a more idyllic portrait of this tie (e.g., Rory and Lorelai in the *Gilmore Girls*, Carol and Maude in *Maude*) whereas other illustrations take on the mother-daughter struggle of holding on and letting go, a tension that characterizes their relationship from birth until death (e.g., *Terms of Endearment*, *Anywhere But Here*, *Spanglish*, *The Joy Luck Club*, *Stella Dallas*). Collectively, however, scholarship and popular artifacts about maternal relating unmistakably illustrate the powerful emotions mothers and daughters feel for one another and continue to experience together during their lifetime.

These portrayals also demonstrate the significance of *communication* in how mothers and daughter relate (or not) to one another. As linguist Dr. Deborah Tannen (2006) asserted, "For girls and women, talk is the glue that holds a relationship together and the explosive that can blow it apart. That's why you can think you're having a perfectly amiable chat, then suddenly find yourself wounded by the shrapnel from an exploded conversation."

In her best seller, *"You're Wearing THAT?" Understanding Mothers and Daughters in Conversation* (2006), Tannen examines how mother-daughter talk creates a relationship that is both "perilous and precious" to the livelihood of women. Their interactions mark their closeness but also their separation.

Researchers have asserted that communication is tied to how this connection evolves. Although mothers and daughters struggle with understanding one another and maintaining their complex dynamic, many experience a special closeness that persists across social classes and generational differences, one that is naturally tied to their shared roles as women in family (Fischer, 1986). It has long been argued that, in comparison with other kin bonds, the mother-daughter relationship has the highest potential for emotional bonding and connectedness (Fischer, 1986, 1991).

In the fields of human communication, family studies, and human development, several texts are perhaps "authorities" on this maternal bond and demonstrate the critical role communication plays in how this relationship develops across time. In the landmark research presented in *Linked Lives: Adult Mothers and Their Daughters*, sociologist Dr. Lucy Rose Fischer (1986) uncovers an honest exposé of how mothers and daughters foster their connection across the life course. In talking to hundreds of women, she captured their increasing intimacy as daughters mature and mothers reevaluate their bond. In particular, she highlighted the daughter's developmental milestones such as getting married, becoming a mother herself, or serving as her mother's caretaker.

Aging scholar Dr. Karen Fingerman's (2003) *Mothers and Their Adult Daughters: Mixed Emotions, Enduring Bonds* explored this growth further by narrowing in on conflict behavior during one particular transition—as daughters enter midlife and their mothers enter old age. Although mothers and daughters may become incredibly close, they can still get under each other's skin. Fingerman's work revealed how an intergenerational dynamic (termed developmental schism) contributes to tension. Given that our needs in life are driven by where we are developmentally in the life span, mothers and daughters may experience tension because of their divergent developmental needs. They will always be from different generations or age cohorts. Yet she also found that, by later life, this may contribute to their ability to become incredibly skilled at conflict management.

Family communication researcher Dr. Michelle Miller-Day (2004) extended Fischer's and Fingerman's research in *Communication Among Grandmothers, Mothers, and Adult Daughters: A Qualitative Study of Maternal Relationships*. She offers one of the only multigenerational examinations of maternal bonds. Miller-Day's research heightened our understanding of how mothers and daughters develop communication patterns, ways or norms of communicating, which can persist across generations of families. In illustrating grandmother-mother-daughter bond development, she also highlighted the dialectical struggles they incur across time, such as managing privacy and openness or being both powerful and powerless. Her award-winning research demonstrates that some maternal communication patterns are even linked to unhealthy outcomes, including disordered eating behavior and drug and alcohol abuse (see necessary convergence communication theory) (e.g., Miller-Day & Fisher, 2008).

As the abovementioned scholarship and popular culture demonstrate, a life-span, developmental lens is useful in understanding how mothers and daughters connect and divide throughout their relational history. A developmental perspective that concentrates on turning points is particularly helpful in appreciating difficulties that can ensue because of abrupt changes (like cancer) and how mother-daughter interaction plays a central role in adaptation and resilience. Transitions, or *turning points*, are important focal points in understanding human behavior across the life span (Baxter & Bullis, 1986).

Turning points are sometimes narrowly described as life-changing events that affect a family's environment or an individual alone. In actuality, turning points are long-term or multiple processes of change that transform a family and its individual members (Cowan, 1991). At times these changes are considered "normative" or stressors we expect as a natural part of aging and maturity (e.g., becoming an adult, getting married, becoming a parent). In other instances, turning points are characterized as "non-normative." These unpredictable stressors are not considered an expected part of the life cycle (e.g., divorce, death early in the life span, a life-threatening illness) (see Segrin & Flora, 2011, for a review on normative and non-normative transitions). Both normative and non-normative transitions alter individuals' sense of self, assumptive world, and behavior. These events also lead to relational adjustments and are moments that eventually redefine family bonds (Baxter & Bullis, 1986).

The communicative behavior that individuals enact to adjust to these changes affects the nature of their transitional experiences. For instance, families may react differently to a cancer diagnosis. According to renowned cancer researchers, "Some families will react to cancer as a frightening crisis best met with a conspiracy of silence; in others, families consciously make themselves extended agents of the patient and medical care system; and there are all shades in between" (Baider & Kaplan De-Noor, 2000, p. xiii).

How family members communicate in response to transitions or turning points such as a cancer diagnosis will, in part, drive their perceptions of how it impacted their individual and relational lives. In light of this, turning points are an important phenomenon of study. They are exemplars of family change that scholars can focus on to better appreciate the importance of interpersonal communication in human survival.

TURNING POINTS AND MOTHER-DAUGHTER COMMUNICATION

Turning points shape mothers' and daughters' linked lives. They lead to relational changes in boundaries, roles, behavior, and intimacy. Moreover, mothers and daughters often jointly take on the challenges of transitions. Cowan (1991) states that when encountering transitions, "The individual, couple, or family must adopt new strategies, skills, and patterns of behavior to solve new problems" (p. 17). Hence, mother-daughter communication is essential to adjusting to turning points competently. A plethora of developmental research illustrates how mothers and daughters bond across time and how their communication shapes the nature of their transitional experiences (Fischer, 1986, 1991; La Sorsa & Fodor, 1990; Miller-Day, 2004).

For instance, a commonly studied normative turning point, the daughter's transition to adolescence, is a time period fraught with issues of autonomy and separation (La Sorsa & Fodor, 1990). Daughters encounter a dialectical struggle between wanting their mother's nurturing presence and needing independence so that they can cultivate a sense of self separate from their mother, a developmental task vital to their health (Hershberg, 2006; Kaufman, 1999). At the same time, the mother must learn to grapple with her daughter's new desire for separation from her and may even feel threatened as she sees her daughter becoming independent and needing her less (Hershberg, 2006). Research since the Women's Movement ascertains that this transitional experience and associated developmental tasks of identity formation (for both mother and daughter) may be further complicated now that contemporary mothers and daughters have more options than traditional woman roles of mother and wife (La Sorsa & Fodor, 1990). Typically, this transitional period is characterized by negative communication, including tense interactions, frequent conflict, and even emotional distance (Fisher, 2005; La Sorsa & Fodor, 1990). Although mothers and daughters experience variant degrees of this challenge, it is likely that these features of communication intensify the difficulty of this transition.

As daughters transition into adulthood, however, how mothers and daughters relate is often redefined. Mothers view daughters' independence more positively or an expected feature of becoming an adult, and daughters often experience a relational shift in how they view their mother, referred to as "seeing the woman behind the role" (Miller-Day, 2004) or "filial comprehending" (Nydegger, 1991). Because of this turning point, they may begin to develop a more egalitarian friendship bond (Fisher, 2004; Fisher & Miller-Day 2006; Miller-Day, 2004). This extends further when daughters marry or become mothers. Their shared role as women in the family or "kin keepers" and increased maturity often bind them closer together (Fischer, 1986; Fisher, 2004; Miller-Day, 2004). Their relationship moves from "role-complement to role-colleague (as mother–mother)" (Miller-Day, Fisher, & Stube, 2013, p. 8). As their understanding of one another increases through these transitional moments, they may alter their communication by becoming more open. This communicative adjustment allows mothers and daughters to become a more intimate presence in each other's lives. Although the struggle with autonomy is a lifelong defining feature of this bond and sometimes returns in full force when a daughter assumes caretaking responsibilities for her aging mother, mothers and daughters seem more competent in managing the stressful changes as they mature. Sheehan and Donorfio (2002) discovered that during mid- and later life, women often alter their communication in ways to maintain acceptance and tolerance. This communicative adjustment ultimately enhances their relational closeness (Fischer, 1986).

When mothers and daughters face such changes—whether they be stressful in nature or not, expected or unexpected—they must be ready to alter their communicative behavior. What worked before in their relationship may not work in their new circumstances. While these normative turning points are defining features of how this maternal bond evolves across time, mothers and daughters can also encounter more traumatic changes (non-normative stressors) or family crises such as divorce or remarriage, death, financial struggles, and illnesses such as breast cancer (Fisher, 2004; Miller-Day, 2004).

In my own research on mother-daughter relational development, breast cancer consistently emerged as a turning point that altered their bond, ways of relating, and, ultimately, communication (Fisher, 2004, 2005; Fisher & Lucas, 2006; Fisher & Miller-Day, 2006). Women who have shared with me their own stories of breast cancer have often asked me what led me to do this research. One reason I give them is that breast cancer kept coming up in any mother-daughter study I was involved in, regardless of the topic or issue at hand. It was clearly a salient issue to mothers and daughters. It was also a turning point I had heard my own mother talk about countless times since I was a child. My mother is the youngest of eight. When she was just a teenager in the 1960s, her oldest sibling and sister, Rose, was diagnosed with the disease in her 30s. At the time, Rose was a mother of four young daughters. She died not long after her diagnosis when she was only 36 years old. My mother has shared with me many memories about this profound loss and the impact it had on the entire family and especially the women in Rose's life—her four daughters, her five sisters including my mother, and my grandmother or Rose's mother. I recall my mother sharing how concerned Rose was for her own daughters and how my grandmother was forever changed after they lost her daughter Rose. The long-lasting impact of breast cancer on Rose's family continues today. Thankfully, although none of Rose's sisters, daughters, or granddaughters has ever encountered the disease themselves, they continue to remember her in many beautiful ways. All three generations of women have joined together in cancer advocacy walks to honor Rose (see p. viii, and Figures 1.1 and 1.2). Rose's daughters also began a tradition of honoring their mother by giving their first-born daughter the middle name "Rose," a loving ritual that some of Rose's granddaughters (as well as a grandson) have continued when naming their own first-born daughters.

CONNECTING BREAST CANCER, MOTHERS, AND DAUGHTERS

Using a developmental lens, one can appreciate the long-lasting, intense impact that breast cancer has on the lives of mothers and daughters. Although how mothers and daughters communicatively cope with the turning point of breast cancer has not been given much attention, the transitional nature of this diagnosis has been examined from other perspectives. In Chapter 2, we explore how this research further demonstrates that the diagnosis of breast cancer is a poignant turning point in the lives of mothers and daughters.

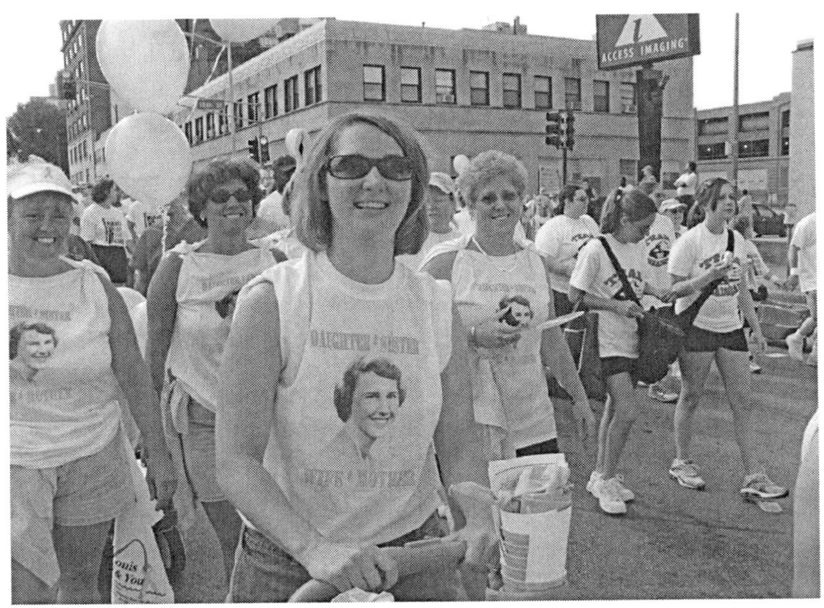

Fig. 1.1. From left to right, Rose's daughters Laura and Carla, Rose's granddaughter, Melissa, and Rose's daughters Diane and Yvonne walking in the 2006 St. Louis Race for the Cure in memory of Rose. Photo: Dan Foust.

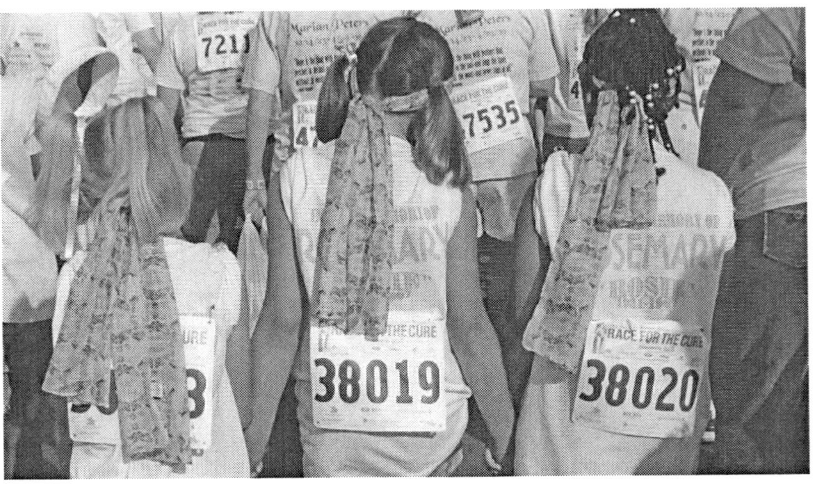

Fig. 1.2. Rose's granddaughter and great-granddaughters. Photo: Dan Foust.

2

BREAST CANCER

A Shared Mother-Daughter Turning Point

My mom says,
*"I didn't go through this. **We** did"*
*It's like **our** thing.*
Daughter of a Diagnosed Mother

The transitional nature of breast cancer has largely been studied as an individual or a woman experience. Indeed, once women are diagnosed with breast cancer, they experience drastic individual changes. Among other things, they must learn to manage intense and complex emotional, psychological changes. Typical experienced emotions include increased anger or sadness, loss of control, feelings of helplessness, increased anxiety and depression, struggles with self-esteem and identity, as well as feelings of betrayal (see Spira & Kenemore, 2000, for a review). Although women of different ages share some of the same psychological manifestations, their age at diagnosis partly determines the individual challenges they face. Oktay and Walter (1991) reported that women diagnosed in their 20s struggle more with anxiety about their future, particularly their ability to have children and form intimate relationships. In contrast, women diagnosed in midlife are concerned with self-reliance and, when they have children, how they are faring. Finally, women diagnosed in later life tend to struggle more with depression and despair in comparison with women in other age groups.

Although women's personal lives are transformed by cancer, their interpersonal lives are greatly altered as well. Spira and Kenemore (2000) observed that, "the closer others are to the patient, the more likely they are to feel that their life is changed" (p. 174). This is true for women's mothers and daughters. Unlike other kin relationships, after a diagnosis, mothers and daughters must both face personal risk and, concurrently, want to support one another (Berlin, 2008). The importance of mother-daughter communication after diagnosis is even more heightened when reviewing research that shows how mothers and daughters share this transition socially, psychologically, and physiologically.

MIRRORED SOCIAL, PSYCHOLOGICAL, AND PHYSIOLOGICAL CHANGES

Research shows that after a woman is diagnosed, their mother-daughter relationship changes (Burles, 2006). Burles determined that some mothers and daughters experience a role reversal. This shift occurs as daughters and mothers take on new roles and responsibilities. For instance, daughters sometimes assume maternal responsibilities such as child care and housework after their mother is diagnosed. Some daughters even take on a more leadership role in the family by becoming the acting parent to younger siblings. In addition to changing roles in the family, the nature of how they relate to one another emotionally can change. After a diagnosis, daughters may provide social support to their mothers and "mother" them for the first time in their bond. Ultimately, breast cancer can result in increased responsibilities for daughters as well as a more mature mother-daughter bond (Oktay, 2005).

Oktay and Walter (1991) noted that these relational changes can be helpful but also difficult. For instance, aging mothers sometimes feel daughters try to take over control, which can result in a power struggle. Mothers with younger daughters may feel that their daughters are not ready to serve in a supportive role to them. Some mothers describe daughters behaving in a distressed manner (withdrawing, becoming angry or sad) when they disclose to them, which suggests that this role reversal is sensitive and not always healthy (Fisher et al., 2014). How these mothers and daughters communicate is critical to how they negotiate these social changes.

The shared nature of breast cancer in the mother-daughter bond is evident on a psychological level as well. Mothers and daughters face a dual battle: They fear for themselves and each other. Daughters of diagnosed women experience a chronic fear of developing the disease themselves and, at the same time, fear recurrence or progression for their mothers. Kenen, Ardern-Jones, and Eeles (2003) assert that like their diagnosed mothers, daughters ultimately live with this psychological "chronic risk." A few select studies have indicated that this shared experience of chronic risk can lead to negative psychological health outcomes. For instance, Boyer et al. (2002) examined the psychological states of women diagnosed with breast cancer and of their adolescent, young-adult, midlife, and later-life daughters (ages 15–71, average age 40). They reported that the patients at times experienced posttraumatic stress disorder (PTSD) symptoms because of their diagnosis and treatment. In these cases, their daughters also exhibited the same PTSD symptoms as their mothers.

Cohen et al. (2002) and Cohen and Pollack (2005) demonstrated that these mirrored psychological changes are also linked to physiological effects. They collected psychological and biological data from adult daughters (ages 20–45) of diagnosed women, their mothers, and a control group of healthy daughters (whose mothers were not diagnosed). Like Kenen et al. (2003), Cohen et al. (2002) found that mothers' and daughters' joint experience appears to be most saliently linked with their shared psychological "chronic risk" distress. When daughters were aware of their increased risk of developing cancer, they displayed higher emotional distress and elevated levels of stress hormones. Moreover, these daughters had higher psychological distress in comparison with daughters of healthy (nondiagnosed) mothers of comparable age and education level. Cohen and Pollack (2005) extended these findings by showing that diagnosed mothers' psychological distress was highly correlated with daughters' psychological distress, particularly when the mother had an advanced stage of the disease. They also determined that these daughters have impaired immune functions and higher levels of stress hormones, which were associated with both their own and their mother's psychological distress. In addition, they found links to social aspects of their collective disease coping. Daughters' perceptions of caregiver burden and frequency of time spent with their mother were also linked to the daughters' psychological stress.

This research supports Oktay's (2005) notion that all daughters of diagnosed moms are "survivors" as well. Her NCI-funded research illustrates the long-term nature of survival of developmentally diverse daughters regardless of whether their diagnosed mothers survived or died. All daughters face major familial changes, worry about their own survival, and experience mental health challenges (although more prominently when a daughter loses her mother). Interestingly, popular culture reiterates this shared experience by suggesting that daughters of varying ages experience anxiety as a result of their mother's diagnosis. In journalist Laurie Tarkan's (1999) book, *My Mother My Breast: Daughters Face Their Mothers'*

Cancer, daughters reveal their own fears and concerns and admit repressing them while their mothers battle the disease so that they are focused on their mother's well-being. Tarkan, who lost her own mother when she was just 11, spoke with other daughters to detail the effects of witnessing a mother's disease. One of her interviewees described how this anxiety has long-lasting effects, saying, "I was paranoid. Any time I got sick, I thought it was cancer." Co-written by a diagnosed mom and her daughter, the book *It's Not About You: A Mother and Daughter's Journey* parallels this discussion (Daniel, Cieszinski, & Biank, 2007). Daniel, the mother, felt unprepared for the impact her disease had on her daughter (Cieszinski) and what her daughter had to go through. They wrote this book together, along with the help of Biank (a licensed social worker and therapist) to aid future mothers and daughters. They especially highlight the need for daughters to dispel their fears and anxieties.

Rarely, if ever, have these studies or books been discussed collectively. In doing so, it is both intriguing and alarming how critical the mother-daughter connection is to a woman's breast cancer experience. In addition to sharing the transition socially, psychologically, and physiologically, research suggests that the shared nature of this turning point persists across the life span and family generations. In particular, personal and familial risk is at the center of women's experiences (Wiggs, 2011). After a diagnosis, mothers and daughters must wrestle with how to minimize each other's future risk *and* how to talk about it.

JOINTLY FACING RISK ACROSS THE LIFE SPAN

According to the American Cancer Society (ACS), just having a mother with breast cancer approximately doubles a daughter's risk of developing the disease during her lifetime. It makes sense then that diagnosed women worry about their daughters, and daughters worry about their futures. For families with a breast cancer history, this united concern for one another is heightened and transmits across generational boundaries.

Many women who are at "elevated risk" for breast cancer (meaning they have a pronounced family history of the disease) seek genetic counseling about breast cancer susceptibility (BRCA) prior to undergoing genetic testing that ascertains whether they carry the gene mutation associated with increased risk (BRCA1 or BRCA2). Women who have a daughter are more likely to do so (Geller, Doksum, Bernhardt, & Metz, 1999). They want to not only better understand their personal risk but identify how it impacts family members (Douglas, Hamilton, & Grubs, 2009; Maloney et al., 2012). Yet even women who receive genetic counseling still describe significant concern and uncertainty about the implications of their genetic profile to their offspring's future (Bylund et al., 2012). Women are especially uncertain about their daughters' disease risks and options for prevention regardless of their daughter's age (Bylund et al., 2012; Fisher et al., 2014; MacDonald, Sarna, Weitzel, & Ferrell, 2010). Relatedly, young-adult daughters of mothers who test positive for the gene mutation also report misconceptions about their risk (Patenaude et al., 2013). In addition, these daughters exhibit high cancer-related stress, which highlights a need for healthy mother-daughter communication about risk. Patenaude and colleagues' work shows these conversations are difficult but could reduce mothers' worry. Furthermore, Tercyak and colleagues at Georgetown Lombardi Comprehensive Cancer Center show that disclosing to young daughters about risk (particularly after testing positive for BRCA1/2) is challenging for mothers, but many do so believing the benefits outweigh the risks (Patenaude et al., 2013; Tercyak et al., 2013). They note that these families would benefit from interventions to help mothers navigate such conversations.

Recent research demonstrates that it is critical for mothers to talk to their daughters about health promotion with regard to cancer because mothers can influence their daughters' health promotion behavior across the life span, including during adulthood. Although mothers with a family history of the disease are more likely to provide daughters with advice on prevention practices such as self-exams (e.g., Kratzke, Vilchis, & Amatya, 2013), mothers play a critical role in helping ensure daughters engage in such practices across adulthood. Sinicrope et al. (2009) examined the advice-receiving experiences of more than 2,000 adult daughters in later life. According to the daughters, mothers rarely (only 9% of this sample) provided them with advice about screening behavior (e.g., getting mammograms, exams, etc.). Yet daughters who received such advice tended to follow it (89%). This was especially the case when daughters had a mother or first-degree relative with breast cancer. In addition, Mosavel's work has shown that a reversal in influence is possible in that daughters may also impact their mothers' cancer screening behavior (e.g., Mosavel, 2012; Mosavel & Genderson, 2013).

For mothers and daughters, talking about risk and prevention is undoubtedly difficult. Clinicians and researchers in the Department of Psychiatry and Behavioral Sciences at one of the world's leading cancer centers, Memorial Sloan-Kettering Cancer Center (MSK), have perhaps led some of the first research on this issue. I was invited to work with them on research pertaining to elevated risk women several years ago. In our collaborative research, we have found that during genetic counseling, mothers describe to clinicians uncertainty about disease risk (their own and their daughters') and future cancer screening (Bylund et al., 2012). Mothers are quite concerned and uncertain about how to communicate such cancer-related information to their daughters (Bylund et al., 2012). They describe a challenging "balancing act" of how much to share and when so as not to cause the daughter stress. Mothers express difficulty talking to their daughters about their own risk, their daughter's risk, health promotion or cancer screening, the mother's risk of death and emotional concerns, and physical changes from treatment (Bylund et al., 2012; Fisher et al., 2014). They describe these conversations as especially challenging and, as such, warrant a mix of communication strategies on the mother's part (e.g., asking questions and using humor) that attend to a daughter's individual characteristics (e.g., age, personality, behavioral cues of discomfort, or readiness to talk) (Fisher et al., 2014).

While less studied, this mother-daughter connection for families of elevated risk or high risk (testing positive for a BRCA mutation) is not missed in popular culture. Sarah Gabriel (2010) profiles the genetic legacy of testing positive and the impact this has on family dynamics for generations to come in *Eating Pomegranates*. She recalls a childhood of losing her own mother to the disease (who died when she was only 42), dealing with her own diagnosis as an adult, and difficulties talking with her two young daughters about how her disease experience affected them. She described this, saying,

> From my most painful experience [losing her own mother young], and from any number of books I have read, I know that you cannot shield children from life, that worse things may result if you think you can. But I know no other way to do it. I refuse to have them spend their childhood in fear. I refuse to allow cancer to take their childhood away from them. . . . "You can ask me any questions you like," I trill endlessly to the children during chemotherapy and for months afterward. "You must feel free to ask me anything." . . . But when it comes to mind, am I ready for her? (p. 243)

Celebrities have also shared their mother-daughter breast cancer stories with the world. Well-known actresses Christina Applegate and Angelina Jolie made headlines in recent years sharing their experiences of familial risk. Both women tested positive for the BRCA1 gene mutation and had double mastectomies in their 30s to minimize their increased risk. Applegate herself is a survivor of the disease and her mother a repeat survivor. Jolie's mother had breast cancer and died of ovarian cancer, as did her grandmother. She also lost an aunt to breast cancer. After having her breasts removed, Jolie reflected on her decision making and medical experience in an op-ed piece in the *New York Times*, telling the impact on multiple generations of family. She described talking to her children about her mother:

> I find myself trying to explain the illness that took her away from us. They have asked if the same could happen to me. I have always told them not to worry but the truth is I carry a "faulty" gene.

Applegate talked about her connection with her mother after having both her breasts removed as a preemptive measure to minimize recurrence:

> She's been sort of this quiet warrior in the back and has been a great support, and just telling me that I was going to be okay. And I knew I was going to be okay. I've watched her. I've watched her have a mastectomy, and then I've watched her go through two years of chemotherapy and eight surgeries and a hysterectomy. I've watched this woman survive both those things. So, for me, there was always that sense that I was going to be okay, no matter what.

When celebrities such as Jolie and Applegate share their experiences with the world so candidly, the media covers it widely, and the general public perks up. Referred to recently as the "Angelina Jolie Effect," disclosures such as theirs have an impact on women's health behavior. According to the National Society of Genetic Counselors, Jolie's disclosure resulted in a marked increase in genetic testing at treatment centers across the country. The same phenomenon was reported abroad: The London Breast Institute claimed a 67% increase. The United Kingdom also saw a surge of women requesting double mastectomies, possibly even when it would not be a necessary preemptive tactic. In essence, when celebrity women share their stories, we listen, and society's awareness of the disease expands, often having influential effects on our health behavior. The same approach—capturing, hearing, and listening to women's authentic narratives—can and should be used to expand our understanding of the familial nature of the disease and influence the way in which we cope with cancer.

The research and popular culture presented in this chapter paint a narrative of breast cancer that is situated within the mother-daughter relationship, and many of these issues that tie mother-daughter communication to breast cancer are far-reaching and long-lasting. However, one issue given less attention or rarely tackled is the nature of how they cope together after a diagnosis or how they might communicate in ways that are both helpful and unhelpful to their disease adjustment. Their interaction, as noted, is central to patients' ability to do this, and yet women and their mother/daughter receive little to no guidance in oncology care as to how to proceed. Rarely are women's mothers and daughters invited by practitioners to their appointments. Given this, mothers' and daughters' coping needs would be better served with information about how to communicatively cope in healthy ways.

MOVING FORWARD: ATTENDING TO THE MOTHER-DAUGHTER JOURNEY WITH BREAST CANCER

My research is an initial step in this agenda. The research presented in the remainder of this book was conducted with two goals in mind. As I discussed in the Introduction, due to incredible advocacy movements in recent decades, breast cancer has become a widely discussed issue in modern society. However, as Richard Suinn (1999) advocated during his tenure as president of the American Psychological Association (APA), we also need to increase public awareness about the role that psychosocial factors play in cancer care. We now need to see the face of family in oncology care more consistently or, for women with breast cancer, an appreciation of the importance of their mother-daughter communication to their well-being.

Thus, the first goal of my research focused on effecting change in patients' health care and expanding societal perceptions of the role of family by demonstrating a need for kin communication to be integrated into patients' care. My second goal was to capture the quality of such kin communication. Ultimately, I sought to enrich mothers' and daughters' coping by ascertaining how they communicate in ways that function adaptively and maladaptively. In essence, to teach mothers and daughters healthy coping behavior or the healing potential of their mother-daughter communication, it is important to illustrate how their behavior may function in healthy and unhealthy ways. By doing this, we can use women's shared stories to develop psychosocial services, education, and interventions to enhance their communication as they communally cope.

In Part II of this book, I explore the healing potential of mother-daughter communication by first presenting the study framework needed to achieve these goals. While a focus on mother-daughter communication in the breast cancer coping context is warranted, so too is one framed by theory. Public health policymakers and scholars argue that theoretical knowledge is needed to create efficacious interventions or services that can help mothers and daughters learn how to cope in healthy ways (Dean, 1996; Michie & Abraham, 2004). Furthermore, a theoretical argument would help advocate for integrating family communication into oncology care.

I begin in Chapter 3 by presenting behaviorally focused health and medical fields of practice and research to demonstrate the need and value of a biopsychosocial approach to care, particularly one that recognizes the role of family in cancer-related stress and coping. In Chapter 4, I extend this perspective and argue for a life-span theoretical lens framing my research that places communication as central to survival, thereby addressing the first goal. This theoretical perspective also highlights the type of communication behavior that might be most critical to mothers' and daughters' healthy coping. I describe these behaviors in the cancer context and attend to the second goal in Chapter 5.

Part II

THE HEALING POTENTIAL OF MOTHER-DAUGHTER COMMUNICATION WHEN COPING WITH BREAST CANCER ACROSS THE LIFE SPAN

3

A BIOPSYCHOSOCIAL PERSPECTIVE

Connecting Family Communication, Health, and Adaptation

Behavioral medicine is the interdisciplinary field concerned with the development of behavioral and biomedical science knowledge and techniques relevant to the understanding of health and illness and the application of this knowledge and these techniques to prevention, diagnosis, treatment, and rehabilitation.
(Schwartz & Weiss, 1978a, 1978b; see also Matarazzo, 1980)

As is certainly evidenced by mothers' and daughters' experiences with breast cancer, this disease is not merely an individual encounter or a biological phenomenon. Rather, illness is socially embedded within the family environment, making kin central to the healing process. Not all oncology care is approached from such a psychosocial perspective. Rather, health care emphasizes a biomedical model, meaning a focus on the individual alone and one's biological and physical aspects of health and illness. Many medical practitioners and scholars have called for a more *biopsychosocial* or *biobehavioral* approach to care, one that integrates patients' social world or family support system with their psychological and physical wellness.

Initiated officially in the 1970s as a branch of the medical field, behavioral medicine highlights the interdisciplinary nature of illness and health and by the late 1980s integrated a focus on the importance of family (Turk & Kerns, 1985). Health psychology also emerged in the late 1970s as a distinct branch of psychology, and both fields are sometimes referred to synonymously as biobehavioral health. In response to behaviorally focused health research rapidly expanding, in 1995, Congress established the Office of Behavioral and Social Sciences Research (OBSSR) within the realm of the National Institutes of Health (NIH) to recognize the significant role of social interaction and behavior in our health and illness experiences. OBSSR serves to encourage behavioral and social scientific research to augment our understanding of disease. Collectively, these more contemporary perspectives recognize what leading life-span, health communication scholars have long argued: "The interpersonal communication that fuels our social world is as essential to our survival as any biological or physical process that keeps us alive" (Hummert, Nussbaum, & Weismann, 1994, p. 3).

Moreover, from a basic family systems theoretical perspective, we know that family cannot be extracted from our health and illness experiences. As one of the founding and leading scholars of family communication, Dr. Kathleen Galvin, explained with colleague and genetic counselor Mary-Anne Young,

> When viewed as a system, families are dynamic, influenced by the ongoing development of family members and their relationships with each other. Ongoing fluctuations occur as every family member affects the other and is in turn affected by them. . . . Family systems foster the exchange of resources such as information and support, . . . influence action among family members and can change or evolve as a function of these actions. . . . According to a family systems approach, all illness influences, and is influenced by, the family members who interpret and manage interactions about the illness. (Galvin & Young, 2010, pp. 103–104)

Family is a pivotal part of patients' coping and survivorship. Although rarely discussed in communication scholarship, theoretically grounded research emerging from the fields of behavioral medicine, health psychology, and biobehavioral health have been instrumental in advocating for the integration of family into patient care. Health fields and practice grounded in this approach highlight the critical role that family behavior plays in wellness and establishes a call for more communication-focused research to improve the health of families in our society.

MERGING HEALTH, FAMILY, AND COMMUNICATION IN HEALTH DISCIPLINES AND PRACTICE

In the early 1990s, renowned psychiatrist Dr. John Rolland introduced a new treatment model that is grounded in family systems theory and identifies the importance of developmental factors or a life-span perspective. Originally based on his clinical work with more than 500 families, the Family Systems-Illness Model comprehensively illustrates the many issues a family encounters when faced with a serious illness or disability. This model is now internationally recognized as an invaluable framework that considers the entire family unit (or caregiving system) rather than the individual patient as the central unit of care, thereby addressing the psychosocial needs of patients *and* their family members.

Later renamed the Family System Genetic Illness Model to include hereditary or familial risk, Rolland's work recognizes the impact of illness/health on families, that families influence the disease experience, and that families are a primary source of support to patients (see Rolland & Williams, 2005). As such, families play a role in both facilitating and inhibiting healthy coping. Furthermore, Rolland uses a multigenerational life cycle approach to integrate time into our understanding of how families cope with illness. According to Rolland (1994), "the impact of chronic conditions on the patient, well family members, and key caregivers differs, and depends on when an illness strikes in the family and in each member's individual development" (p. 8). Before this model, the developmental aspects of disease and individuals were largely ignored.

A subfield of the therapy discipline and practice supports the stance for a biopsychosocial approach to patients and is aligned with Rolland's work. McDaniel, Hepworth, and Doherty presented their pioneering book in 1992 to introduce the field of medical family therapy. Like Rolland's model, they argue for a more ecological approach to health care that links the health care team, patient, family, and illness and appreciates how interactions among these "systems" affect a patient's treatment and coping. They identify family social support, stress, and coping as critical components to how individuals adapt to and survive life-threatening and chronic illnesses. In their approach, they advocate for integrating pertinent biological concepts into therapy and provide a foundation for collaboration among physicians, therapists, and other health professionals.

Likewise, this focus on family continues with practitioners and scientists in the field of genetic counseling who recognize that "genetic disease affects entire families, not just individual members" (Bylund, Galvin, & Gaff, 2010, p. 3). Gaff (a genetic counselor who has practiced internationally) and Bylund (a behavioral scientist and associate director of Hamad

Medical Corporation's Medical Education in Doha, Qatar, and former director of MSK's Communication Skills Research and Training Laboratory for providers) believe that addressing family communication issues (e.g., who to tell, when to tell, and understanding family dynamics) should be a core role for genetic counseling practice. In their text (*Family Communication About Genetics: Theory and Practice*) in which every chapter is co-written by a practitioner in genetics and a family communication scholar, they also provide encouraging guidance on how this can be facilitated through interdisciplinary team models of care (Gaff, Galvin, & Bylund, 2010; see Gaff & Bylund, 2010).

Although not always integrated into cancer care, a biopsychosocial framework has also been advocated by leading oncologists. Dr. Jeremy Geffen, a medical oncologist and founder and director of the Geffen Cancer Center and Research Institute in Vero Beach, Florida, offers cancer patients and their families a guide in his seven-level program that integrates every dimension of a human being in an effort to beat cancer. He integrates aspects of physical, mental, emotional, and spiritual layers of one's health; merges Eastern and Western medical principles; and highlights the need for patients to have a strong family support network. In his ground-breaking book, *The Journey Through Cancer* (2000), he offers a healing model that attends to both patients' and their families' needs with regard to treatment options and disease information, psychosocial support, alternative and complementary medicine, emotional and cognitive challenges, finding meaning, and spirituality.

As health practitioners and scientists continue to adopt a biopsychosocial lens in health care practice and research, variants of this perspective offer patients a new treatment approach or more holistic care. At the same time, this research emphasizes the need for communication scholarship that identifies the critical role that family interaction plays in health and illness or the intersection of family and health communication (see Galvin & Braithwaite, 2014). Recent texts by communication scholars support this idea. Dickson and Webb's (2012) *Communication for Families in Crisis: Theories, Research, & Strategies* and Miller-Day's (2011) *Family Communication, Connections, and Health Transitions: Going Through This Together* demonstrate the "healing power of communication within families as they faced a myriad of crises," in particular health challenges such as postpartum depression, dementia, and infertility (Dickson & Webb, 2012, p. 5). These edited books present ground-breaking scholarship that depicts how family dynamics are both challenged and altered after illness, highlighting how complex issues such as interdependence and stigma further complicate members' coping. Accordingly, these works are suggestive that patients' and their families' communication needs must be at the center of health care.

Studies need to address how kin interaction affects patients' wellness across the entire cancer trajectory. Communication scholars are apt for capturing how communication in the family can function both adaptively and maladaptively. With this in mind, communication research could serve as the bedrock for developing psychosocial services, education, and therapies for families coping with breast cancer.

COMMUNICATION RESEARCH: A FOUNDATION FOR PSYCHOSOCIAL INTERVENTION-MAKING

Leading behavioral medicine researchers Anderson, Kiecolt-Glaser, and Glaser (1999) advocate that interventions must attend to cancer patients' health behavior given the links between behavior and health effects such as psychological distress and immunity. Unfortunately, interventions, policies, and education to support families are still not widely included in traditional cancer care (Rolland & Williams, 2005). Nearly a decade ago, Rolland advocated at the National Cancer Institute (NCI) and American Cancer Society (ACS) bi-annual meeting on survivorship that families direly need a "psychosocial map" to learn healthy communication central to coping and health promotion behavior that minimizes disease risk.

The lack of a psychosocial map or guidance for families still exists today and is of concern as families admit not knowing how to be supportive. Patients also report unhelpful kin communication, which is likely tied to members' not knowing what to say or do or not being aware that what they are doing and saying is not necessarily helpful to their loved one's adjustment and stress management. Communication competence in coping is something families gain across the life span as they increase their social experiences (Pecchioni et al., 2005). Moreover, after a life-threatening transition such as cancer, families must learn to adjust their behavior (Cowan, 1991) and often need help learning how to do so in a healthy manner.

The health industry needs to expand its approach to cancer care by integrating family communication into the process on a more consistent basis. A theoretically grounded approach is essential to increase the likelihood of ever effecting changes in policy and practice in the health care industry. Health intervention scholars (Dean, 1996; Michie & Abraham, 2004) claim that studies must incorporate theory to generate the type of knowledge needed to create interventions and ensure their efficacy in helping families. According to Michie and Abraham (2004), theories provide an explanation for "psychological processes accounting for the initiation, redirection or cessation of behaviour achieved by the intervention" (p. 33).

As the NCI advocates, a biopsychosocial, patient-centered approach better appreciates patients' need for healthy kin communication (Arora,

Street, Epstein, & Butow, 2009). However, knowledge for interventions must be appropriately focused to ensure families' needs are met and, therefore, that services will be efficacious in helping them cope. A theoretical framework that establishes connections among family communication, cancer, and adaptation is important. In Chapter 4, I explore this idea further by unpacking currently used theoretical frameworks in stress and coping research. I also offer a psychosocial theory that can serve as a lens that merges our understandings of family communication, coping, and health and, as such, is apt for producing knowledge rich for intervention-making.

4

THEORETICAL APPROACHES TO FAMILY COPING AND STRESS

Integrating a Psychosocial Life-Span Lens

> *The absence of theory and effective theory building are serious weaknesses of much of the existing research available for the policy making process for improving the health of populations.*
> (Dean, 1996, p. 20)

Stress and cancer go hand in hand. Across the disease trajectory, diagnosed individuals and their families encounter a number of stressors or "discrete life events or transitions that have an impact upon the family unit and produce, or have the potential to produce, change in the family social system" (Olson, Lavee, & McCubbin, 1988, p. 19). Thus, when one thinks of stress, a negative feeling or connotation is often associated. However, not all stressors and stress are bad. Rather, how a family *responds* to that life-changing event partly influences how they experience distress as a result of the stressor at hand.

A number of theoretical perspectives have entered into studies of how families respond to stressors and cope with stress (see Afifi & Nussbaum, 2006; Maguire, 2012; Segrin & Flora, 2011, for excellent reviews of stress and coping frameworks). While family communication is key to that response, thereby mediating how we adapt to challenging events, how we conceptualize family communication or its role in managing stress and health varies. To establish an argument that communication is *central* to survival (and add to the argument that family communication be integrated into cancer care), the theoretical lens guiding the research must conceptualize family communication in the same way. In reviewing currently used stress and coping theories, this issue comes to the forefront.

STRESS AND COPING THEORIES

Most of the widely used theoretical frameworks portray coping in terms of cognitive functioning or characterize communication in the family as a resource. A common approach is to conceptualize an individual's entire social network as a resource critical to one's ability to cope and adjust. Frequently used stress and coping theories such as the buffering hypothesis (Kaniasty & Norris, 1997) and support deterioration model (Barrera, 1989) suggest that individuals' social networks affect their adjustment to stressful events. These perspectives are useful in recognizing that individuals' access to social networks (i.e., friends, family, loved ones) affect how they adjust to stressful changes (Afifi & Nussbaum, 2006). In other words, these theories allow us to see how one's social network is a resource utilized in coping.

Other scholars have approached stress and coping developmentally. Life-span attachment theory and intergenerational solidarity theory indicate how family attachment is instrumental in helping families cope with difficult changes (Bowlby, 1979; Cicirelli, 1983, 1991). These theories posit that some families adjust to stress better because they have developed closer, stronger attachments across time (Bowlby, 1979) or because they have established relational rules and norms about solidarity (i.e., when to be there for one another) (e.g., Bengston & Harootyan, 1994). Similarly, from developmental frameworks, then, closeness, relational norms, and attachment are considered resources in family coping.

Still other theories are useful in considering the entire family system, such as is done from the perspective of "communal coping." Scholars drawing on this lens examine how families cope as a whole or collectively (Afifi, Hutchinson, & Krouse, 2006; Lyons, Mickelson, Sullivan, & Coyne, 1998; Wolf, 2009). Communal coping is purportedly an effective way to deal with stressors because family members combine their resources and problem-solving skills to adjust collectively. Essentially, they view the crisis at hand as "their" issue (not one individual family member's crisis). As a result of their combined efforts, their coping is more effective. One of the most valuable and widely tested models within this approach, McCubbin and Patterson's (1982) Double ABC-X Model of Family Adjustment and Adaptation, even includes a communication component. Based originally on Hill's (1949, 1958) research on families coping with separation during World War II and the ABC-X Theory of Family Crisis, this model examines the adaptation process that families go through from pre- to post-crisis, noting that family communication like social support is a resource used to handle the stressor. Similarly, Olson's (1993) Circumplex Model conceptualizes communication as a segment of family behavior that can facilitate adaptability to stress, particularly cohesion.

According to these and the bulk of perspectives taken in stress and coping research, family communication is a *resource* for coping. Afifi and Nussbaum (2006) identify this trend and suggest that, although this is true and certainly helpful in understanding families' adjustment, the communication is also a *means* of coping. To highlight the critical role that family communication plays in cancer coping and survivorship, a theory is needed that prioritizes it as central to our survival across the life span. In essence, the communication component of coping in the family needs to be approached a bit more intricately. A life-span perspective of communicative behavior provides researchers with the means to achieve this.

A LIFE-SPAN PERSPECTIVE OF COMMUNICATION AND HEALTH

In his ground-breaking book published in the late 1980s, *Life-Span Communication: Normative Processes*, Nussbaum (1989) was the revolutionary communication scholar to propose that researchers integrate a life-span approach to more aptly attend to the complexities of human communication across the entirety of our lives (Nussbaum, 1989; Pecchioni et al., 2005). Nussbaum's life-span perspective of communication emphasizes "real-world issues" and is grounded in Baltes, Reese, and Nesselroade's (1988) life-span developmental psychology or the "description, explanation, and modification (optimization) of intraindividual change in behavior across the life span and interindividual differences (and similarities) in intraindividual change" (p. 4). Today, Nussbaum's wealth of texts and research offer the field a foundation on which to examine communication as a developmental phenomenon. According to Nussbaum and his former students, who are now also renowned life-span communication scholars, Dr. Loretta Pecchioni and Dr. Kevin Wright, "communication is not a single, time-irrelevant object" (Pecchioni et al., 2005, p. 10). Rather,

> Communication is a primary skill to be mastered so that meanings can be transferred effectively and efficiently. . . . Communication is best viewed as a flow of events across time rather than a static occurrence. . . . Communication events are continuously unfolding and impacted by a

> wide range of individual characteristics and factors as well as previous experiences of those involved in the event. . . . As the communication process unfolds within human interaction, changes occur on numerous levels that may be manifested in different ways at various points in the life span. . . . An individual's capacity to communicate must continuously develop for that individual to master his or her environment and to interact effectively throughout the transitions, adaptations, and new challenges that arise over the life span. (pp. 10–11)

Life-span perspectives propose that individuals are constantly adapting to their changing environment (Baltes, 1987), and their social lives are a critical component of their adaptability (Carstensen, 1991, 1992; Nussbaum, 1989). According to Lang and Carstensen (1994), "consistent with life-span theory is the proposition that adaptation is not simply reactive. Rather, individuals maintain a proactive role in constructing social environments such that they match and enhance individual competencies" (p. 316).

Studies grounded in Carstensen's (1991, 1992) psychosocial life-span framework, socioemotional selectivity theory (SST), further suggest that communication partner choice matters. Whom one chooses to interact with is one element of how an individual constructs his or her social environment to adapt in a manner that enhances life. SST is a life-span theory that provides a lens in which we can examine how we prioritize interaction in certain bonds (such as family) during specific circumstances (i.e., cancer) in an effort to maximize well-being, adaptability, and, ultimately, survival. Although it has yet to be done, numerous leading communication scholars have indicated that SST could be particularly useful in aging, health, and family research (e.g., Afifi & Nussbaum, 2006; Nussbaum, Pecchioni, Robinson, & Thompson, 2000; Segrin, 2006).

SOCIOEMOTIONAL SELECTIVITY THEORY: FAMILY COMMUNICATION AS ADAPTIVE BEHAVIOR

Socioemotional selectivity theory (SST) suggests that communication is central to one's survival, particularly during life-threatening changes. Communication allows a person to fulfill goals critical to his or her well-being and adjustment across the life span. Moreover, this theory predicts that individuals carefully choose with whom to interact to attain these goals.

The theory assumes the following: (a) interaction is necessary for survival, (b) humans interact on the basis of personal goals, and (c) people select goals prior to interacting. According to Carstensen, Isaacowitz, and Charles (1999),

> Knowledge- and emotion-related goals together comprise an essential constellation of goals that motivates social behavior throughout life. . . . Socioemotional selectivity theory addresses the role of time in predicting the goals that people pursue and the social partners they seek to fulfill them . . . in order to adapt effectively to their particular circumstances. (pp. 166–167)

Basically, SST posits that time drives human motivation (i.e., goals) and considers this cognitive influence in predicting how people adapt their communicative behavior to achieve their goals.

In understanding how women cope with breast cancer, according to SST, after diagnosis, they may prefer communicating in certain relationships to maximize their ability to achieve goals central for survival. Such interactions are a critical part of their adjustment to the disease and, therefore, survival. The components of SST, as outlined further here, can be aptly applied to an investigation of breast cancer coping and family communication. In exploring the theoretical tenets associated with goals and time, it is also possible to narrow in on aspects of mother-daughter communicative behavior that are important to their adjustment.

Predictions of Goals and Communicative Behavior

According to SST, human motives that are critical to survival direct behavior. Individuals prioritize goals on the basis of perceptions of time (Carstensen et al., 1999). They see time as either limited or unlimited. When one perceives time as unlimited, one also perceives the future as uninhibited. In opposition, when time appears to be limited, the future appears to be constrained. These perceptions of time direct one's prioritization of knowledge- or emotion-focused goals. Individuals perceiving an unlimited future prioritize knowledge-seeking goals because information is a useful resource in the future. In contrast, individuals perceiving a limited future prioritize goals regarding emotional quality of life. They prioritize present-oriented needs because they value their present circumstances more so than their future.

Once goals are prioritized, individuals select social partners with whom to interact to achieve the goals and prioritize communication with partners who best enable them to fulfill these goals (Carstensen et al., 1999). Future-oriented individuals motivated to pursue information interact with any person who can enhance their knowledge of their social and physical world. In contrast, people with a limited time perspective seeking emotional stability are more careful about determining with whom to interact, as not everyone can help them achieve emotionally related goals. Such a person is inclined to seek interaction with individuals with whom he or she already has a strong relational history (e.g., family members) because they have greater perceived potential to satisfy his or her socioemotional needs.

Markers of Time

As noted, an individual's goals and communicative behavior are ultimately based on his or her perception of time. One's perspective of time is typically influenced by one's place in the life cycle. In other words, chronological age determines how much time we perceive we have left in life (Carstensen et al., 1999). Older adults (e.g., age 75) typically view their time left in life as more limited than younger adults (e.g., age 25) (Carstensen, 1992; Carstensen et al., 1999; Lang & Carstensen, 1994). Thus, they prioritize present well-being (rather than the future), and therefore emotional goals, and tend to select close, familiar interactive partners (such as family members) to achieve those goals in opposition to younger adults.

However, one's sense of time can also be affected by life events. According to Carstensen et al. (1999), "endings" are transitional events that are life-threatening in some way and can be encountered at any point in the life span. These events cause people of any age to view time as limited because their end of life appears closer. When this is the case, they reprioritize emotional goals as older adults do and select close interactive partners, such as kin, to adapt to their circumstances. For instance, Carstensen and Fredrickson (1998) explored the impact HIV status can have on young gay men's perception of time and how that, in turn, influenced their prioritization of goals and partner choice. They found that men who were both HIV positive and symptomatic (vs. without disease symptoms) felt increasingly closer to the end of life. They prioritized emotional goals sought via communication with close friends and family.

Conceptualizing Cancer as an "Ending"

Although a cancer diagnosis is a traumatic transition commonly encountered in the family, this major life event has not yet been explored from this theoretical perspective. A diagnosis of cancer is consistent with SST's definition of an ending because individuals coping with cancer experience a temporal shift that leads them to prioritize emotionally salient needs. Compas et al. (1999) note that, although an individual diagnosed with cancer may receive a favorable prognosis, the perception that life is threatened is inevitable for the patient and his or her family. In accordance with SST, cancer patients' and their families' time perspective of the patient's life becomes limited. Moreover, cancer heightens one's emotional needs. This health transition is characterized by overwhelming emotions that can result in distress, anxiety, and even depression (David, 1999). Even though the experience of cancer may vary (e.g., site of malignancy, stage of disease, type of treatment), all cancer patients have similar emotional needs (Helgeson & Cohen, 1999). They most often pursue goals associated with self-esteem, perceived control, feelings regarding the future, as well as emotional meaning and processing (Helgeson & Cohen, 1999). Again in accordance with SST, present emotional wellness is prioritized when an individual is diagnosed with cancer.

In addition, interaction is vital to cancer patients' adjustment. Communication within a patient's social support network is a determining factor in whether his or her emotional goals are met (see Kahn & Antonucci, 1980; Thotis, 1985). Cancer patients often seek support via interaction with family members (Helgeson & Cohen, 1999; Mallinger et al., 2006). Perceived emotional support is associated with patients' positive social and emotional adjustment, specifically enhanced role functioning, self-esteem, reduced hostility, and life satisfaction (Jamison, Wellisch, & Pasnau, 1978; Zemore & Shepel, 1989). Emotional support also appears to contribute to better physical health (Ell, Nishimoto, Mediansky, Mantell, & Hamovitch, 1992). When a patient's mental and social health decline, his or her immunity and other biological processes often do as well, resulting in negative health outcomes (Anderson, Kiecolt-Glaser, & Glaser, 1999). Thus, in accord with SST, communication, particularly within kin bonds, appears to be central to patients' adjustment. Moreover, this communication is emotionally focused because of patients' prioritization of present well-being. Thus, breast cancer fits within the framework of SST as an "ending" transitional event that affects women's perspective of time, social goals, and, ultimately, communication needs and preferences.

Still, two gaps in the foundational theoretical research exist that need to be addressed prior to establishing the theory's utility in understanding the importance of family communication to cancer coping. Carstensen and colleagues never tested the theory to ascertain individuals' communication partner preferences specifically for family bonds. They only focused on whether the tie was a familiar versus an unfamiliar bond. They conceptualized "familiar partners" in their testing procedures as inclusive of family, friends, and other close loved ones but never separated out their findings by relationship type within each group. To fill the first gap, the theory must be tested and extended to identify a preference specifically for communicating with *familial* partners.

PRIORITIZING FAMILY COMMUNICATION IN ADAPTATION AND SURVIVAL

Carstensen and colleagues have used a list of 18 potential communication partners that includes both novel and familiar partners (see Carstensen & Fredrickson, 1998; Fredrickson & Carstensen, 1990). Of the familiar partners, several family bonds are used (e.g., sibling, younger relative, immediate family). However, when scholars use this list to examine participants' communication partner preferences, they do not distinguish between family and familiar partners and only distinguish between familiar and nonfamiliar/novel partners. As a result, familial ties are confounded with familiarity in Carstensen's procedures. Fredrickson and Carstensen recognize this limitation in their research and even call for scholarship that differentiates familiar and familial social relationships.

In this vein, I sought to establish a specific preference for family communication using SST assumptions. Conducted in collaboration with Dr. Jon Nussbaum, we used the same partner list as Carstensen and colleagues with a modified survey measure and examined women's partner preferences as they age across the life span (see Fisher & Nussbaum, 2014). According to SST, it is likely that as women age, they will increasingly prioritize communication with family bonds as a means of maximizing their survival and well-being. More than 300 healthy women representing young, middle, and later adulthood participated. Our results supported our prediction and showed a moderately strong relationship ($V = .406$) between partner preference and age: As healthy women age, they increasingly prioritize communication with family partners as opposed to other close or familiar relationships. Younger women exhibit significantly different interactive partner preferences based on their age. Only 43.2% of young adult women reported a kin member as their first partner choice in comparison with 76.5% of women in midlife and 87.5% of women in later life.

We were able to extend the theory and demonstrate that not only do we prioritize communication in familiar bonds as our perspective of time left in life becomes more and more constrained, we increasingly favor communication with family given the potential for these partners to help us attain emotionally salient goals critical to adaptation and survival. The second gap to fill then is to examine this in an unhealthy context or investigate whether breast cancer functions as an "ending," according to SST assumptions, thereby leading women to prioritize family communication to enhance their coping abilities.

STUDY PHASE I: ESTABLISHING THE IMPORTANCE OF FAMILY COMMUNICATION AFTER CANCER

As noted, SST posits that regardless of age, individuals experiencing an ending will select close, familiar partners (often family members) to achieve emotion-focused goals (see Carstensen & Fredrickson, 1998; Fredrickson & Carstensen, 1990). It is likely that a breast cancer diagnosis fits SST's conceptualization of such a time-altering event, and given psycho-oncology literature, it is likely that when individuals are diagnosed with cancer, they prefer family members as opposed to other close, familiar communication partners. Still, this possibility remains to be established and presents an opportunity in which to extend the theory. By doing so, it is possible to also establish a theoretically tested argument that family communication is central to health when coping with cancer.

Extending SST in this way would contribute to accomplishing the first objective of this research by encouraging the health industry to expand its approach to cancer care by establishing that patients' families are integral to their adjustment and well-being. By using SST, it is possible to test whether patients prioritize communication in their family bonds as a function of their adaptability. By extending SST, a theoretical argument for family communication as central to survival can be established.

THE NEXT STEP: CAPTURING THE NATURE OR QUALITY OF THE ADAPTIVE INTERACTION

To move toward the second objective of the foundational research, the conversation must advance forward and address what this communication looks like. As I articulated in this chapter, the tenets of SST postulate the type of communication most central to women's coping and survival. They prioritize communication that allows them to fulfill emotionally focused goals—needs tied to their emotional well-being and coping. In Chapter 5, I establish a link between the perspective of SST and current psycho-oncology research. In doing this, I reveal a more centralized focus on how mothers and daughters communicatively adapt to breast cancer by identifying types of behavior and contextual factors critical to their coping.

5

COPING WITH CANCER

Openness, Avoidance, and Emotional Support

Psychosocial programs for cancer patients should be able to assist focused groups on a solutions-based approach to emotional issues [that] teach communication skills [and] support networking skills.
Former American Psychological Association (APA) President,
Dr. Richard M. Suinn

To help families learn to communicatively adjust in healthy ways, the adaptive and maladaptive functioning of how they interact—the manner and quality of their communication—must be captured and explained. Communication is critical to understanding how families respond to the strenuous turning point of cancer and how they ultimately may emerge strengthened and resilient. As was illustrated in Chapter 4, a socioemotional selectivity theoretical lens suggests that individuals facing a life-threatening change like cancer will prioritize goals central to their present emotional well-being in order to adjust in a manner that maximizes survival. Cancer-related research supports this idea. In the last two decades, psycho-oncology researchers have become more concerned with how family communication can affect patients' socioemotional well-being as they adjust to the disease (Edwards & Clark, 2004; Ell, 1996; Manne, Dougherty, Veach, & Kless, 1999; Manne et al., 2005). Although most of this scholarship centers on one kin bond (married couples), the research indicates that three types of emotionally focused behavior are especially critical to how families cope: open communication, avoidance, and emotional social support.

OPENNESS AND AVOIDANCE IN CANCER COPING

In general, open communication is the disclosure of feelings, thoughts, and information whereas avoidance refers to evading cancer-related talk. Such interaction reflects the ability to talk openly about cancer with a loved one, as well as the patient's partner's willingness to engage in such a discussion. Hilton (1994), Figueiredo, Fries, and Ingram (2004), and Porter, Keefe, Hurwitz, and Faber (2005) classify open communication as patients' and partners' disclosures to each other concerning their fears, emotional issues, and doubts associated with cancer. Scholars use a variety of terms to represent such communication phenomena, and openness is often juxtaposed with avoidant communication to highlight how these behaviors impact a patient's disease adjustment differently. For instance, Hagedoorn et al. (2000) compare "active engagement" (openly talking about concerns and feelings associated with cancer) with "protective buffering" (hiding feelings or concealing information). Depending on the context, individuals are motivated to disclose or avoid communication for many reasons (e.g., to enhance relational closeness) (see Goldsmith, Miller, & Caughlin, 2008, for a review). Likewise, different factors predict individuals' openness and avoidance (e.g., fear of stigma).

The potential outcomes of individuals' open or avoidant communication are indicative of whether the behavior of interest functions in adaptive or maladaptive ways. In particular, it is important to consider how these behaviors impact patients' and their families' relational, psychological, and physical well-being. A large amount of scholarship indicates that open communication functions adaptively for couples adjusting to cancer (Boehmer & Clark, 2001; Hilton, 1994; Mallinger et al., 2006; Porter et al., 2005; Rosenberg et al., 2002). This behavior is reportedly the most satisfying form of communication for married couples, even up to a year past diagnosis (Hilton, 1994). Research involving communication interventions shows similar findings. When men with prostate cancer receive an intervention that stimulates open communication in a supportive relationship, they have better pain control and care management over time in comparison with men who do not receive such an intervention (Rosenberg et al., 2002). These findings are also evident in general studies of disclosure, avoidance, and adjustment. Gross and Levenson (1997) noted that selective social interactions likely play a role in not only minimizing emotional distress but in diminishing psychophysiological arousal associated with negative affect. In addition, Pennebaker's (1995, 1997, 2003) widely cited work reveals that disclosure is critical in healing and regulating emotion when coping with difficult experiences. He has shown that emotional expression, or disclosure, positively affects health by substantially improving psychosomatic conditions (Berry & Pennebaker, 1998; Davison & Pennebaker, 1996).

In opposition to openness, avoidant behavior is largely deemed an unhealthy coping approach and typically associated with poor health outcomes. Research relating to avoidance in personal relationships further suggests this behavior is maladaptive, in that avoidance is predictive of relational dissatisfaction (Caughlin & Golish, 2002). Cancer-related research supports this notion. Diagnosed individuals who engage in avoidant communication tend to experience poorer relationship functioning, increased psychological distress, and poorer adjustment to cancer in comparison with patients communicating openly (Boehmer & Clark, 2001; Kershaw et al., 2004; Mallinger et al., 2006; Porter et al., 2005).

This association is also true for breast cancer patients specifically. Those patients who engage in more topic avoidance when coping tend to have higher levels of depression and anxiety (Donovan-Kicken & Caughlin, 2011). Avoiding topics is also linked to women seeking less emotional support and feelings of self-blame. In turn these outcomes are associated with higher levels of psychological distress. Women's physical health and cancer progression are also of concern. When diagnosed women engage in avoidant coping between the time they are diagnosed and their surgery, their physical health is compromised. For instance, they can experience disrupted everyday rest/activity rhythms (e.g., daytime sedentariness) (Dedert et al., 2012). This is particularly concerning because tumor growth is regulated by circadian rhythms and, as such, considered a prognostic of early death in metastatic breast cancer patients.

Cancer-related research characterizes openness as healthy communication and avoidance as unhealthy behavior. It is not unreasonable to state that Western or North American research clearly favors open communication and its adaptive functioning. The research cited earlier provides sound health-related reasons for this contention. Yet it also reflects a more general bias in scientific research to publish positive (statistically significant) results (Goldsmith et al., 2008). Although scholarship inconsistent with this partiality for open communication exists, it is much less abundant, particularly in the health-related research. Some research suggests that avoidant communication may function adaptively as well. Two ongoing programs of communication research (Baxter and Montgomery's dialectics and Petronio's communication privacy management) indicate that *both* open communication and avoidance can be beneficial to individuals' relational well-being (see Baxter & Montgomery, 1996; Petronio, 2002). Relatedly,

Pederson and Valanis (1998) found that not all families benefit from open communication when adjusting to cancer.

What is perhaps most important to recognize is that openness and avoidant communication are complex phenomena, and neither is all good or all bad. It is too simple to just advise patients and their families to talk openly (vs. avoiding discussions). Moreover, the research is somewhat flawed. Scientists often evaluate open and closed communication quite generally, ignoring conversational factors such as the issue patients are coping with, what relationship they are communicating in, or where in the cancer trajectory they are (e.g., during treatment or as they transition to survivorship). To better understand how openness and avoidance can function both adaptively and maladaptively for mothers and daughters, the outcomes of these behaviors depend on a variety of such factors or the *context* of communication. Context is a critical, multidimensional influential factor in individuals' interactive experiences. Scholars can view context broadly or narrowly and, depending on the lens, may focus on how sociocultural, episodic, and/or relational contexts affect communicative behavior outcomes (Goldsmith, 2004). By considering context, researchers engage in a more ecological approach to understanding health behavior and illness and move further than one level of analysis by recognizing the interconnected nature of various factors involved (see Sallis, Owen, & Fisher, 2008, for a review of ecological approaches to health promotion; see Bronfenbrenner, 1979, for an ecological approach to family behavior).

According to leading communication scholar Goldsmith (2004), "The notion that effective communication must be adapted to a *situation* to overcome constraints and obstacles is foundational to the study of communication (Clark & Delia, 1979)" (p. 23). Thus, the outcomes of avoidance and openness depend on situational factors; still, context is surprisingly absent in research. Goldsmith and colleagues (2008) identify a variety of contextual factors that conceivably determine whether open communication and avoidance function positively or negatively. Three factors (the topic of disclosure/avoidance, reason for disclosure/avoidance, and cohort/age diversity) may be particularly useful in understanding how mothers and daughters use open communication and avoidance to adjust to breast cancer. In addition, families establish patterns of communication across their life span or what might be considered expected behavior or norms of openness or avoidance in their culture. Thus, their relational history with regard to openness is an important dynamic to explore.

Topics to Disclose or Avoid

Various topics present different challenges. Accordingly, a given topic could elicit diverse responses from various interactive partners. The types of cancer-related topics that mothers and daughters may openly communicate about or avoid include death, future plans, treatment and its side effects, bodily changes, sexual functioning, daily life, and feelings and fears. Goldsmith et al. (2008) suggest that some of these topics are likely more challenging to communicate openly about than others in certain kin bonds, and cancer-related research supports this idea. Women report that talking about medical aspects of the disease is easiest (Pistrang & Barker, 1992), whereas talking about mortality is most challenging or talked about the least (Lewis & Deal, 1995). Moreover, the relationship matters: Some women describe disclosures being the most difficult in spousal relationships (Pistrang & Barker, 1992). As noted previously, elevated risk mothers of adolescent daughters, most of whom were also survivors, characterized talking about a range of cancer-related topics as difficult, including risk, health promotion behavior, death, and bodily changes (Fisher et al., 2014).

These findings suggest that not only are some topics more difficult to disclose, but diagnosed women may prefer to only discuss particular topics with certain relational partners. Moreover, juggling openness and privacy is a difficult dilemma that already characterizes the nature of mother-daughter communication across their entire relational history (Fisher & Miller-Day, 2006; Miller-Day, 2004). What women feel comfortable openly discussing as it pertains to breast cancer in this bond likely varies. This may also depend on what role (mother or daughter) the patient plays in the relationship. Another factor to consider is why women are motivated to share some aspects of the cancer experience with their mother or daughter and avoid other topics.

Motivation to Disclose or Avoid

One's motivation for disclosure or avoidance can play an important role in whether the behavior is helpful to women's disease coping. In their review of the literature, Goldsmith et al. (2008) observe that some individuals openly communicate to coordinate support and reassure each other that they can deal with whatever happens in the future. In addition, people may disclose concerns to reaffirm closeness or commitment to one another. Thus, openness for these reasons likely functions adaptively. Numerous reasons for not disclosing or avoiding conversations also exist: protecting one's partner; reluctance to express emotions; maintain privacy, hope, or normalcy; avoid unnecessary talk; and preserve identity or relational characteristics (Goldsmith et al., 2008). Mothers and daughters likely have various motives for avoiding or disclosing certain topics, which may impact whether the behavior is adaptive.

In addition, the adaptive coping potential for both of these contextual factors is likely linked to where mothers and daughters are in the life span.

As such, women's age or developmental diversity is an important factor to consider.

Cohort and Age Diversity

Generational cohorts differ in their evaluation of open communication in the family (Suitor & Pillemer, 2000). Older generations grew up in a more closed environment. In other words, they experienced a culture in which they were not encouraged to express their feelings and concerns freely. This norm certainly speaks to the silencing culture of cancer that many older generations experienced. In comparison, younger generations have grown up in a social world that more often encourages and accepts openness. This has resulted in younger generations having different open communication preferences than older generations. General relational research supports this. Couples married in more recent decades prefer open, frank discussions in opposition to married couples of older generations (Zietlow & Sillars, 1988). Research demonstrates that such differences influence open communication in the parent-child bond as well. For instance, aging mothers are less likely to be open about problems in comparison with their adult children (Suitor & Pillemer, 2000). Additionally, adult daughters tend to communicate more overtly than their aging mothers (Fingerman, 2003; Mottram, 2003).

While age affects open communicative behavior, it also influences individuals' cancer experiences. Age impacts how much couples coping with cancer actually talk about adjustment-related issues (Hilton, 1994; Northouse, 1994). Older patients and their spouses tend to discuss cancer less than younger patients and their spouses (Hilton, 1994). Moreover, age affects women's breast cancer-related concerns, which are potential topics of discussion (Oktay & Walter, 1991). This too is in line with Rolland's family treatment model (see Chapter 3), which purports that one's developmental place in life affects how a member experiences an illness.

Collectively, these previously mentioned, often overlooked factors also highlight diversity in a family environment. Another often disregarded feature of family behavior is the fact that families establish patterns of communicating across their history. They establish norms and rules about appropriate behavior that define their unique familial environments. As such, these patterns play a role in whether behaviors such as openness and avoidance are established "norms" in a family's culture and, therefore, suggest that these behaviors may function in both adaptive and maladaptive (unhealthy) ways.

Family Communication Patterns of Openness and Avoidance

Family communication patterns or ways of communicating are developed across time. These patterns are partly defined by how open or closed families are and suggest that there is not one way to functionally behave. Family Communication Patterns (FCP) theory further supports the notion that families co-create ways of communicating and, according to the theorists, "is not based on the assumption that there is only one functional way to communicate. . . . [Rather] different families function well by employing different types of behavior" (Koerner & Fitzpatrick, 2006, p. 61).

FCP theory is a particularly well-known and established theory used in family communication scholarship but not yet utilized in cancer coping research (Fitzpatrick & Ritchie, 1994; see Koerner & Fitzpatrick, 2006, for a review of the theory). Grounded in McLeod and Chaffee's (1972) original model, FCP theory emphasizes that openness is a significant aspect of how individuals communicate as a family unit. Conversation orientation refers to the degree to which a family encourages and fosters an environment of open expression of variant ideas and beliefs. Families high on this dimension tend to be highly interactive without many limitations in disclosure and share more in activities and emotions.

While not yet tested in a cancer context, FCP theory may help interventionists not only identify families that need assistance coping more openly but be a tool for researchers to better link health outcomes with behavioral family environments that cultivate openness or avoidance. Given the abundance of research that suggests openness is tied to better health outcomes, one may assume that families coping with cancer who are also historically more open (high on the conversation orientation) would experience better health outcomes as opposed to those families who tend to be more avoidant (low on the dimension). Still, this factor (a family history of communicating openly or not) has yet to be examined in psycho-oncology research.

In summary, the topic of disclosure/avoidance and reasons for doing so, along with women's age and whether their families already foster openness in their environment, all influence families' openness and avoidant behavior and partially determine whether the communication will function adaptively in women's adjustment to cancer. In addition to openness, social support is another form of adaptive family communication frequently studied. Still, in reviewing the current literature, questions remain about how this communication can function both adaptively and maladaptively in mothers' and daughters' adjustment.

ENACTED SOCIAL SUPPORT

Social support is a broad construct that can refer to many social phenomena and processes (Goldsmith, 2004). In general, family social support is an interactional transaction in which members express support to one another. Across disciplines, there are a number of social support taxonomies (e.g., Cobb, 1976; House, 1981; Krishnasamy, 1996) and conceptualizations (e.g., Caplan, 1974; House, 1981; Weiss, 1974). One conceptualization, *enacted support*, is a frequent object of interest among communication scholars. Enacted support refers to what people say and do for each other and how such behavior can enhance well-being (Goldsmith, 2004). According to notable social support scholar Dr. Brant Burleson and colleagues, social support behavior, in part, defines healthy family communication (Burleson, Albrecht, Sarason, & Goldsmith, 1994).

Unfortunately, across disciplines, researchers interested in social support rarely capture actual communicative behavior. Although social support is conceptualized as an interactive phenomenon, seldom do scholars actually measure social support by focusing on communication. According to Dr. Daena Goldsmith (2004), renowned expert in social support communication,

> Interactions in which individuals discuss their problems and communicate various types of support are a central feature of the multifaceted social support construct and yet these interactive processes are among the least studied components of social support. (p. 4)

Instead, most studies assess support-related interactions between patients and loved ones by means of self-report surveys and tend to focus on phenomena other than communicative behavior (Manne & Schnoll, 2001). For instance, scholars use scales to determine patients' perceptions of available support (Bloom & Kessler, 1994; Klemm, 1994), the number of social contacts or size of their social network (Bloom, 1982; Funch & Marshall, 1983), the number of people they feel they can talk to about their concerns (Northouse, 1994), and the number and quality of their relationships (Koopman, Hermanson, Diamond, Angell, & Spiegel, 1998). How people communicatively enact support does not receive as much attention.

In understanding how social support can function adaptively in families' coping, the most insightful research is that in which the support behavior is connected to the recipient's perception of whether it was helpful. This is most valuable in understanding how families' communicative behavior can function both adaptively and maladaptively in their adjustment to cancer. In such scholarship, three types of support are typically the foci: informational, instrumental, and emotional. Scholars then attempt to link the type of support with patients' quality of life (House, 1981; House & Kahn, 1985; Kahn & Antonucci, 1980; Thotis, 1985). *Informational support* consists of giving or receiving information to advise or guide a loved one. In a cancer context, these types of interactions can alleviate patients' confusion about their illness. These behaviors also correlate with less depression (see Helgeson & Cohen, 1999). *Instrumental support* involves the provision of tangible resources such as transportation, finances, or assistance with household tasks. Such interactions can improve patients' well-being by balancing their sense of loss of control. Financial support, for instance, has been associated with better physical recovery (Funch & Mettlin, 1982).

From a socioemotional selectivity theory perspective, the third type is especially heightened in breast cancer coping:

> *Emotional support* involves the verbal and nonverbal communication of caring and concern. It includes listening, "being there," empathizing, reassuring, and comforting. Emotional support can help to restore self-esteem or reduce feelings of personal inadequacy by communicating to the patient that he or she is valued and loved. It can also permit the expression of feelings that may reduce distress. Emotional support can lead to greater attention to and improvement of interpersonal relationships, thus providing some purpose or meaning for the disease experience. (Helgeson & Cohen, 1999, p. 54)

This form is arguably most important in patients' adjustment (Helgeson & Cohen, 1999), a view supported using a socioemotional selectivity theoretical perspective as well. Emotional support includes a variety of caring behaviors, such as empathizing, listening, reassuring, reciprocity, affect, and comforting. Family emotional support reportedly contributes to better psychological functioning, including less depression (Edwards & Clark, 2004), less mood disturbance (Figueiredo et al., 2004), and better overall adjustment (Manne et al., 1999; Pistrang & Barker, 1992). Some studies have shown that certain types of emotional behavior (e.g., affect and reciprocity) are associated with better quality of life outcomes (e.g., decreased depression) (Primomo, Yates, & Woods, 1990).

Once scholars categorize communication into one of these three types of support, they ascertain whether they are helpful or unhelpful (or perceived by the patient as supportive or unsupportive). In doing this, scholars are able to examine the adaptive functioning of communication. For instance, both Dunkel-Schetter (1984) and Dakof and Taylor (1990) determined that cancer patients perceive emotional support (specifically showing love, concern, understanding, reassurance, encouragement, empathy, affection, and physical presence) as more helpful in their adjustment than informational or instrumental support. In addition, patients have reported that when loved ones enact certain types of emotionally supportive behavior (e.g., unrelenting optimism), the individual to whom the support was directed may find it to be upsetting (Peters-Golden, 1982). Therefore, in this context, the behavior may constitute an unhelpful or unsupportive communicative response. Patients in some studies have found other emotionally supportive behaviors unhelpful in their adjustment (e.g., minimizing the problem, forced cheerfulness, avoidance/withdrawal, insensitive comments, and being told not to worry) (Dakof & Taylor, 1990; Dunkel-Schetter, 1984).

Classifying behavior as either helpful or unhelpful is common among scholars studying enacted support across contexts (see Goldsmith, 2004). The behavior has been an object of studies in various challenging circumstances, including cancer, HIV or AIDS, bereavement, depression, work stress, rheumatic diseases, chronic conditions, and divorce. The research is abundant and potentially revealing. Goldsmith (2004) compiled these findings and created a typology consisting of two lists of communicative behaviors that individuals use to adjust to difficult life events. One list consists of the most commonly reported helpful enacted support, and the second list is comprised of unhelpful behavior. This research and Goldsmith's typology contributed to a better understanding of the adaptive functioning of communication during transitions. Nonetheless, this research has some limitations.

To begin with, some of the "helpful" forms of enacted support on Goldsmith's (2004) list are somewhat specific (e.g., expressed affection). Other listed categories of behavior are more abstract and could present a variety of specific acts (e.g., engaged in coping). This limitation is evident in both lists. In addition, many of the same types of behavior listed as "helpful" also appear in the "unhelpful" list (e.g., showing concern). Goldsmith identifies these restrictions and characterizes the descriptions of behavior in this typology as abstract, general, and contradictory. She explains this outcome in relation to limitations in the existing literature from which the typology was created. She notes that one significant limitation is that scholars consistently overlook the context in which the support is enacted. As was previously mentioned, context influences behavioral outcomes (Goldsmith et al., 2008). Thus, this disregard for context is problematic.

APPRECIATING THE CONTEXT OF ENACTED EMOTIONAL SOCIAL SUPPORT

Pioneering and leading communication researchers of social support, Drs. Terrance Albrecht and Daena Goldsmith (2003), assert that social, relational, physical, and temporal aspects of context are critical considerations in understanding supportive communication and its respective individual and relational outcomes. The context in which people enact such behavior determines, in part, its efficacy. Although recognizing the context in which behavior occurs is constraining and can limit the generalizabilty of the findings, clear individual differences in communication exist, warranting such an approach (Goldsmith et al., 2008). Goldsmith (2004) argues that "studying enacted support within a particular context is necessary if we are to ask and answer questions about meaningful, purposeful action" (p. 45). Without context, the adaptive functioning of these behaviors cannot be fully understood.

Scholars' lapse in considering context may be attributable to the limitations of their methodological approach. Research involving social support often entails use of self-report survey methodology. Hence, researchers begin with preconceived assumptions about the behavior one enacts in any interaction involving social support. Unfortunately, their presumptions are at times artifacts of scales originally created in non-family, non-cancer contexts (e.g., the Barrera [1981] and Barrera, Sandler, & Ramsay [1983] Inventory of Social Support Behaviors [ISSB]). Using such scales to measure social support in response to cancer presumes that the way people communicatively enact and receive support (or how they would describe and make sense of these behaviors) is consistent across contexts. However, among families coping with the life-threatening diagnosis, treatment, and survival of cancer, the enactment, description, and interpretation of that social support may be rather different.

Capturing context is an enormous task. As noted previously, context can be viewed through a broad or narrow lens, and scholars may choose from among numerous potential foci. Closer examination of the current scholarship suggests that two specific factors (the relationship in which support is communicated and individuals' cohort/age) warrant closer consideration in future research and are particularly appropriate for this examination of mother-daughter emotional support.

Relational Diversity

The relationship in which support is enacted affects whether it functions adaptively. Patients report that different forms of enacted support behavior can be helpful when received from one type of interactive partner (e.g., doctor) but not another (e.g., family member). Rose's (1990) findings suggest that patients tend to prefer informational support from medical professionals and one specific type of emotional support (ventilation) from family. Some emotional support behavior (e.g., affect) may only be effective in enhancing patients' well-being when expressed by family partners (Primomo et al., 1990). Researchers have also revealed that some types of emotional support (e.g., minimizing the problem) appear to be unhelpful when family or friends, as opposed to other relational partners, express them (Rowland, 1989; Wortman & Lehman, 1985). Such findings suggest that the potential adaptive functioning of social support depends on the person with whom the patient is interacting. Certain types of support may only be desirable (and efficacious in adjusting) when particular relational partners enact it.

Although these studies demonstrate that the relational context matters, scholars still fail to appreciate fully the bond as a factor of influence. When they have assessed the bond as a source of variance, they have done so in a broad manner. In studies, patients typically only identify the type of relationship the support came from (e.g., friend, family member, or medical professional) rather than specify the relationship (e.g., marital, sibling, or parent-child) about which they are reporting (e.g., see Rowland, 1989). In addition, when researchers actually do examine communication in specific family bonds, they tend to concern themselves primarily with martial communication. It is likely that this narrow approach stems from the fact that spouses are widely considered the key sources of support for cancer patients (Manne & Schnoll, 2001; Pistrang & Barker, 1998). The fact that other family bonds play a role in patients' adjustment has been largely a matter of neglect. This oversight is disconcerting when one considers that mothers and daughters are reportedly important in breast cancer patients' adjustment (Burles, 2006; Oktay & Walter, 1991; Spira & Kenemore, 2000). Likewise, a patient's age or place in the life course is often given less attention.

Cohort and Age Diversity

As discussed previously, communication is a developmental phenomenon (Nussbaum & Friedrich, 2005; Nussbaum, Pecchioni, Baringer, & Kundrat, 2002; Nussbaum, Pecchioni, Robinson, & Thompson, 2000). Individuals communicate differently and have distinct communication needs as a function of where they are in the life course (Pecchioni et al., 2005). For instance, older individuals often exhibit more competent communication in comparison with younger individuals because they have more life experiences. Age differences also are in evidence in communicative behavior attributable to cohort variability (Segrin, 2003; Zietlow & Sillars, 1988). Zietlow and Sillars (1988) explain that because individuals in different generations grew up in contrasting sociocultural contexts, they exhibit different communication preferences. Segrin (2003) found this also to be true of support communication preferences. In comparison with older generations, younger people's well-being appears to depend more on receiving social support from diverse sources. Finally, age is a factor in women's breast cancer experiences. Age at diagnosis drives cancer-related concerns (Oktay & Walter, 1991), which in turn alters their support needs. Again this need to appreciate developmental diversity matches Rolland's life cycle approach to understanding illness, in which he also prioritizes social support in the family. Collectively, this research suggests that age/human development/cohort variability is determinant as a factor of influence in individuals' support communicative experiences that would appear to require further examination.

MOTHER-DAUGHTER EMOTIONALLY FOCUSED COMMUNICATION: CAPTURING COPING

Theoretical scholarship using a socioemotional lens and psycho-oncology research both support the belief that women's emotionally focused communication behavior enacted in their family environment is central to their coping and survival. Thus, within this frame, it is important to examine communicative behaviors of openness, avoidance, and emotional support to capture how mothers and daughters adjust to this disease together. As Rolland showed in his family model of health, human development or age is typically ignored in stress and coping research even though it affects the nature of the illness one encounters as well as an individual's coping behavior. Thus, to best attend to mothers' and daughters' needs, it is important to consider their experiences when diagnosed across adulthood or throughout their relational life span.

In Part III of this book, I revisit the study goals and present a mixed-method research design utilized to conduct this research. A mixed-method design is necessary to both extend our conceptualization of family communication as central to survival and vividly describe, in their own words, mothers' and daughters' lived communicative experiences as they cope with breast cancer together. The research inquiries guiding this study are presented in Chapter 6 within the scope of the study framework. In Chapter 7, I introduce the women of the research and show how their stories were captured by mixing paradigms to both extend theory and elicit knowledge for intervention-making. I also introduce an innovative multi-method qualitative design to capture authentic coping narratives that consists of triangulating narrative data from in-depth interviews, longitudinal diaries, and diary interviews.

Part III

OVERVIEW OF FOUNDATIONAL STUDY

6

BUILDING THEORY AND CAPTURING COPING NARRATIVES FOR INTERVENTION-MAKING

Theory, research, and practice are interrelated.
(Crosby, Kegler, & DiClemente, 2009)

This theoretically driven foundational study was meant to provide intervention-making knowledge for the creation of psychosocial services and education geared toward providing communication guidance to mothers and daughters in how to adjust to breast cancer in a healthy manner. Ultimately, this research was conducted to enhance mother-daughter communication—or their health behavior and well-being—by providing them with a "psychosocial map" in coping with breast cancer.

This mixed-method, two-phase study was centered around two primary aims: (a) to investigate the significance of family communication to health and survival when adjusting to breast cancer, and (b) to explore how diagnosed women communicatively adjust to the disease in their mother-adult daughter bond to highlight ways in which they can engage in healthy coping specific to their point in the life span. To fully attend to these goals, this foundational study involved women diagnosed across the life span (in young, middle, and later adulthood) as well as their developmentally diverse mothers and daughters.

IMPORTANCE OF FAMILY COMMUNICATION IN WOMEN'S ADJUSTMENT TO BREAST CANCER

Carstensen's (1991, 1992) socioemotional selectivity theory (SST) offers scholars a suitable framework for confirming the importance of family communication in women's adjustment to breast cancer. In previous research, I further extended SST tenets by showing a specific prioritization of communication in family bonds as opposed to any familiar relationship as women age or near the end of the life span (Fisher & Nussbaum, 2014). This paved the way to explore the significance of family bonds in the context of cancer coping.

An SST lens is suggestive that when individuals face a possibly terminal experience, they construct a limited time perspective and give priority to emotionally related goals that are most critical to their healthy adaptation and survival—goals that can only be fulfilled via interaction with close, familiar loved ones, particularly kin. SST suggests that these interactions are critical to individuals' survival and, thus, may provide a theoretical argument to integrate family communication more consistently into oncology care, practice, and interventions.

Although the psycho-oncology literature suggests that diagnosed women prefer kin communication partners, the theory had yet to be tested to affirm this. Also, granted the diagnosis of cancer appears to fit the Carstensen et al. (1999) conceptualization of an "ending," it has yet to be tested as an ending event within the SST framework. This raised the question of whether cancer leads women of any age to prefer communication in kin bonds. Specifically, I explored the following question: How does breast cancer function in women's lives as an ending transition with regard to their preference for kin communication partners, regardless of age?

While testing SST in this regard may lead to a theoretical argument justifying the importance of family communication to healthy adaptation when coping with cancer, it is also important to connect family communication with better health outcomes to demonstrate the central role that family communication plays in healthy cancer coping and survivorship. In line with an SST perspective and psycho-oncology research, emotionally focused behavior is critical to women's coping, particularly openness. Openness tends to be linked to healthier outcomes, whereas the opposite behavior, avoidance, is associated with unhealthy outcomes.

Yet we know, based on research grounded in Family Communication Patterns Theory, that open and avoidant behavioral norms are cultivated in family environments across their history. When families encounter a cancer diagnosis, they are already functioning within familial cultures in which openness is either routinely encouraged or discouraged to some degree. Given cancer-related research today, we may expect that mothers and daughters who tend to already be more open with each other might experience better health outcomes after diagnosis. Still, family studies suggest that because these patterns are cultivated and defined across their relational history, openness and avoidance may function differently for families. This raised the following question: When coping with breast cancer, what health outcomes are associated with mothers and daughters who have an established pattern of openly communicating in their relational history in comparison with those dyads that engage in avoidant coping?

CAPTURING ADAPTIVE MOTHER-DAUGHTER COMMUNICATION

As noted in the second aim, the next step in helping women enhance their mother-daughter coping behavior is to actually capture the *quality* of their interactions or how mothers and daughters cope together. To aid families in improving their communication competence when coping, it is necessary to examine what their communication looks like and how it functions in their adjustment and management of stress associated with this life-threatening transition.

I sought to extend the findings from Phase 1 by illustrating the quality of their interactions or how mothers and daughters communicatively adapt in both healthy and unhealthy ways. Based on SST, emotionally focused behaviors (e.g., openness, avoidance, and emotional support) are particularly important to women's ability to cope with breast cancer and, as such, of primary focus. Moreover, contextual factors such as relationship type, age/human development, and topics and motivation for communication all presumably have something to do with why communication can function in both helpful and unhelpful ways. Thus, the following research inquiries were of particular interest:

- What cancer-related topics do developmentally diverse women diagnosed with breast cancer openly communicate about or avoid in their mother-adult daughter relationship?
- What motivates diagnosed mothers' and daughters' open and avoidant behavior?
- How do developmentally diverse women diagnosed with breast cancer communicatively adapt to breast cancer through enacted emotional support in their mother-daughter bond?
- How do these emotional support behaviors function adaptively or maladaptively in diagnosed women's adjustment?

EXECUTING THE STUDY

In Chapter 7, I introduce the women who participated in this foundational study and the design needed to achieve the goals. While the Phase 1 goal to extend SST to investigate the prioritization of family relationships and mother-daughter openness in human survival warranted an empirical approach, the aim of Phase 2 or the collection of women's real, lived mother-daughter experiences called for a focus on authentic narratives of coping. Therefore, a different, more interpretive lens—one that allowed for vivid illustrations of the context of mother-daughter communication—was essential. The broad life-span framework and embedded theoretical lens (SST) guiding this study supports the philosophy that science should be open to the need to blend or merge multiple paradigms or worldviews and associated methodological approaches (Pecchioni et al., 2005). Thus, a mixed-method design was employed in this research. According to the National Institutes of Health (2011),

> Multi-pronged strategies . . . are critical to effectively tackling today's most pressing public health problems . . . [and] require rigorous data to understand and effectively address these problems. This often requires both quantitative and qualitative data. . . . Mixed methods research combines these methods and capitalizes on the strengths of both.

In the next chapter, I provide an explanation of how I mixed these paradigms. I offer a research design that may prove useful to other social scientists concerned with the complexity of our familial health and illness encounters and who are conducting research with the intention of providing theoretically driven and rich, in-depth knowledge ripe for intervention-making.

7

MIXING METHODS AND PARADIGMS

> *As a methodological movement, mixed methods research is expanding across the social, behavioral, and health sciences. . . . Mixed methods is, simply, best suited for addressing many of today's complex research questions, which require context and outcomes, meaning and trends, and narratives and numbers.*
> (Creswell & Clark, 2007, p. 184)

Although not necessarily a new approach for scientists, recent scholars have centered in on the value and process of conducting mixed-methods research or the employment of both quantitative and qualitative approaches in one study (Morse & Niehaus, 2009). When I first began this research in 2006, I was still surrounded by much debate and, at times, heated discussion and conflict primarily between quantitative versus qualitative researchers and a penchant for conducting studies from one approach, usually prioritizing a quantitative or an empirical lens. Yet today, the appreciation of not only qualitative scholarship but mixed-methods research continues to surpass this constricted, archaic dispute. Fortunately, in recent years, international authorities on health research, such as the National Institutes of Health (NIH) and the Centers for Disease Control and Prevention (CDC), have prioritized knowledge sought via mixed-methods designs as a necessary approach to effectively capture a more comprehensive scientific and humanistic understanding of health and illness. The mixed-methods movement has garnered so much attention and support in the last decade that in late 2010, a team of leading mixed-methods experts was convened by NIH's Office of Behavioral and Social Sciences Research (OBSSR) to develop a "best practices" resource meant to guide NIH investigators on how to conduct, develop, and evaluate research using this approach (this resource is available online at http://obssr.od.nih.gov/mixed_methods_research/).

Several prominent authorities on mixed-methods design (e.g., Drs. John Creswell, Vicki Plano Clark, Janice Morse, Linda Niehaus, and Margarete Sandelowski) offer behavioral scientists invaluable guidance on the components involved or the anatomy of mixed-methods designs, complex decision making when developing such a study, as well as principles for executing rigorous and sound mixed-methods research (see Creswell & Clark, 2007; Morse & Niehaus, 2009; Sandelowski, 2000). While various debates, discussions, and disagreements still abound across these scholars' conversations, collectively their works and guidance helped to inform the design of this mixed-methods family heath behavior study.

This mixed-methods study employed a QUAN + QUAL design, meaning quantitative and qualitative data were concurrently collected and analyzed to understand the important role that mother-daughter communication plays in breast cancer coping. The design used herein best fits Creswell and Clark's (2007) definition of a variation of an embedded mixed-methods design (the correlational model) in that the qualitative findings in Phase 2 help explain relational factors presented in Phase 1. Using survey methodology, the goal of Phase 1 was to demonstrate the significance of family communication to diagnosed women's coping and adjustment (i.e., relationships among women's cancer diagnosis, prioritization of family communication partners, mother-daughter openness patterns, avoidant coping behavior, and health outcomes). The goal of Phase 2 was to then provide the details of these associations by capturing the quality of women's mother-daughter interactions using multiple qualitative methods. In other words, the qualitative findings identify specific communicative coping behaviors (conceptualized as forms of openness, avoidance, and emotional support) and women's perspectives of how such behaviors function adaptively or maladaptively by influencing diagnosed women's wellness at various points in the life span. Additionally, a multi-methods qualitative design was incorporated in Phase 2 of this larger mixed-methods study to allow for the triangulation of data from three interpretive methods (interviews, longitudinal daily diaries, and diary interviews) to further validate findings and extend our understanding of the nature of mother-daughter breast cancer coping across both the human life span and the trajectory of the disease.

Prior to outlining the mixed-methods design and each phase of this study, I provide an introduction of the women who graciously shared their experiences with me and the multiple recruitment methods I engaged to meet these women.

THE PARTICIPANTS: RECRUITING AND MEETING THE MOTHERS AND DAUGHTERS

The study required women diagnosed with breast cancer who had received some sort of treatment (e.g., surgery, radiation, or chemotherapy) within the last 36 months to ensure that their memories and experiences with cancer were still quite salient. To decouple age and time for the testing of SST and ensure developmental diversity was appreciated as a factor in the adaptive potential of mother-daughter coping communication, cross-sectional data were needed, meaning women were recruited to represent three age groups: (a) young adulthood (ages 30–39), (b) middle adulthood (ages 40–56), and (c) later adulthood (ages 57+).[1] Sampling was purposive because predefined groups of women were needed, and proportionality was not the primary concern. Rather, the goal was to include women who could best report on experiences relevant to the research topic (breast cancer and communicative adjustment) during particular points of adulthood across the life span.

Recruitment of Women

Following Institutional Review Board (IRB) approval, various recruitment efforts were used. Women were recruited using a northeastern university's department-based research requirement in which students must complete research credit each semester when enrolled in a capstone course of the university (they are given alternative options so as to not coerce participation). Students with diagnosed mothers were recruited using this approach and asked to inform family members about the study if they qualified to participate. Women were also sought using local paper and online flyer postings with the university newswire, local hospitals and support groups, local cancer clinics, grocery stores, community bulletin boards, and cancer websites.

[1]Additional specific information about the breakdown and characteristics of these developmental periods is provided in the beginning of each chapter in Part V. Middle and later adulthood were altered from typical developmental breakdowns (e.g., ages 40–60 for midlife or ages 60+ for later life) to account for the age distribution of the women recruited.

In addition, several medical institutions on the East Coast agreed to post recruitment flyers in their offices. One breast health and cancer clinic agreed to distribute flyers to newly diagnosed women. Recruitment also occurred in two hospitals based in Pennsylvania. One hospital was a 201-bed acute-care community hospital located in a small rural town. The second hospital was a larger level-1 trauma center with more than 500 beds located just outside a large urban city. Both recruitment efforts required additional IRB approvals. For the smaller rural hospital, recruitment was conducted in collaboration with the hospital's administrative director of the cancer program using mailings to the hospital's support group participants and by posting flyers in the hospital. Recruitment at the larger urban medical center was coordinated with the hospital's women's health clinic and breast imaging via collaboration with the section chief physician, chief radiology technologist, and head nurse and coordinator of breast care services. Information was distributed to physicians, radiology patients, at monthly support group meetings, and on hospital bulletin boards. Collectively, recruitment took nearly a year to complete. Each participant received $25 compensation thanks to funding from local and private grant awards.

Meeting the Women

Although most of the women completing Phase 1 of the study also participated in Phase 2, a few did not participate in both portions. As such, demographic information on the women is provided according to each data set.

For Phase 1, 76 women participated (39 diagnosed women and 37 of their mothers and daughters). Diagnosed women represented the three age groups, although only 39 of the diagnosed women provided demographic information. Of these women, 9 were young adults. Their average age was 34.63 ($SD = 3.34$) and encompassed a range from ages 30 to 39. Another 18 women were in middle adulthood. Their average age was 48.16 ($SD = 3.11$), with a range from ages 42 to 52. Finally, 12 women were in later adulthood. Their age on average was 61.92 ($SD = 4.48$) and ranged from ages 57 to 69. Time since treatment was variable. Some participants were currently in treatment (27.5%), 37.5% had had treatment within the past 12 months, and 35% of women had treatment within 12 to 36 months prior to their participation. They also varied according to stage at diagnosis: 41% had a diagnosis in stages 0 or I, 27.5% in stage II, 25% in stage III, and 5% in stage IV. Four of these women were experiencing a recurrence. Most of their mothers and daughters also participated in Phase 1, in which associations between their communicative behavior and health outcomes were assessed ($N = 37$, 12 mothers and 25 daughters) with an average age of 38.8 years old ($SD = 20.35$).

A total of 35 dyads or 78 women (40 diagnosed and 38 mothers/daughters) participated in Phase 2. Of the 35 mother-daughter dyads, 3 had an additional daughter participate, whereas 5 diagnosed women participated without a partner. Their mothers/adult daughters did not participate for various reasons (e.g., could not be contacted, refused to participate, or the diagnosed woman did not want her to participate). Women represented the three age groups. The middle adulthood age group represented two types of dyads: midlife diagnosed daughters and their mothers and midlife diagnosed mothers and their daughters. Of the diagnosed women, 8 were young adults (all as daughters: *mean* age = 34.62, *SD* = 3.34, age range 30–39), 20 in middle adulthood (13 as mothers: *mean* age = 49.42, *SD* = 2.50, age range 44–52; 7 as daughters: *mean* age = 46.00, *SD* = 3.00, age range 42–51), and 12 in later adulthood (all as mothers: *mean* age = 61.92, *SD* = 4.48, age range 57–69). The remaining 38 women represented the mothers and adult daughters of diagnosed women. Of the mothers or daughters of diagnosed women, 25 were in emerging[2] or young adulthood (all as daughters: *mean* age = 24.74, *SD* = 6.94, age range 18–37), 5 in middle adulthood (4 as mothers and 1 reporting as a daughter: *mean* age = 54.00, *SD* = 2.35, age range 51–56), and 8 in later adulthood (all as mothers: *mean* age = 69.86, *SD* = 7.59, age range 58–83).

These participants represented mostly a Northeastern small, rural community in the United States, although five women were from Canada. Among the participants, 98.7% were White, and 85.3% lived on the East Coast. About half of the women had incomes under $70,000 per year, whereas the other half had greater annual incomes. Half were currently married, 20% single, 10% separated, 10% divorced, and 10% widows. Half the women worked full time, 21.3% worked part time, 16% did not work, and 17.3% were students. Most had a college-level education, with 40% earning a baccalaureate or graduate degree and 41% having an associate's degree or some college credit.[3]

---

[2]Emerging adulthood (ages 18–29) follows adolescence and precedes young adulthood (see Arnett [2000] and Chapter 8 for more distinction between the two developmental periods).

[3]The demographic information specific to each age group of dyads appears in the first results section (findings on openness) to make clear the sociocultural context of women in each age group of mother-daughter dyads.

PHASE 1: MEASURES AND ANALYSIS: THE IMPORTANCE OF FAMILY COMMUNICATION TO HEALTH AFTER A BREAST CANCER DIAGNOSIS

In addition to completing a background questionnaire to collect demographic information, women completed five surveys or questionnaires to examine the critical role of family communication after a cancer diagnosis. To extend socioemotional selectivity theory, diagnosed women completed an SST questionnaire that assessed the prioritization of family communication partners after a breast cancer diagnosis. Diagnosed women and their mother or daughter also completed the Revised Family Communication Patterns (RFCP) scale to provide information about the nature of openness in their mother-daughter relational history and the Impact of Events Scale (IES) to provide information on avoidant coping behavior. Quality of life was also assessed socially, psychologically, and, for diagnosed women only, physically. Social or relational health was measured using a modified version of the Marital Opinion Questionnaire (MOQ). Psychological well-being was examined using the Impact of Events (IES) scale while diagnosed women's physical health was measured using the Functional Assessment of Cancer Therapy–Breast scale (FACT-B).

Family Communication Partner Preference: SST Questionnaire

To test and potentially extend the tenets of socioemotional selectivity theory as a means of heightening the significance of family interaction to cancer coping, procedures used by Carstensen and colleagues (e.g., see Carstensen & Fredrickson, 1998) were slightly modified to create a questionnaire. In their studies, they presented participants with an 18-card set consisting of a potential partner on each card (Carstensen & Fredrickson, 1998). Each description was general so as to apply across ages (e.g., "a younger relative" as opposed to "a grandchild"). Participants identified on the cards with whom they most liked to spend their time. The investigator then divided responses into one of two categories: familiar or novel partners. While the same partner list was used for the current study, this list instead appeared on a questionnaire. This modification ensured that women not residing in the area could participate, thereby increasing the study sample size. Women wrote on the sheet three individuals from the list with whom they most liked to spend their time, in order of preference. Women's first choice responses were grouped into one of two categories: family or nonfamily partners.

Openness: RFCP Scale

The RFCP measure is a 26-item scale (Ritchie & Fitzpatrick, 1990) used to assess two core dimensions of family communication: conversation orientation and conformity orientation. Women were asked to report on communication in their mother-daughter bond only, and scores on the subscale of conversation orientation were evaluated for this study. Language was changed on the scale so that women reported on communication in their mother-daughter bond specifically. Using 15 items, the conversation orientation subscale measures the degree to which a family encourages participation and interaction over a wide variety of topics or how openly a family communicates. Women indicate their agreement (1 *strongly disagree* to 5 *strongly agree*) with statements such as, "We often talk about topics like politics and religion where some persons disagree with others" and "I can tell my mother almost anything." The items were averaged with a higher score indicating a stronger conversation orientation ($M = 3.86$, $SD = .74$, $\alpha = .90$). The internal reliability was comparable to other studies.

Avoidant Coping and Psychological Health: IES Scale

The IES is widely used to measure the impact of a traumatic event on women's intrusive thoughts and avoidant coping responses and is frequently used in evaluating stress after such an event (Horowitz, Wilner, & Alvarez, 1979). As such it can be used to examine both mental distress and avoidant behavior. The questionnaire consists of 15 items that can be revised to specifically address the impact of breast cancer on a woman's well-being and coping behavior. IES was used to assess psychological health and coping on two levels: avoidance and intrusion. Intrusion items included items such as, "Pictures about it popped into my head," "I thought about it when I didn't mean to," and "I had dreams about it." Avoidance items included items such as, "I avoided letting myself get upset when I thought about it or was reminded of it," "I stayed away from reminders of it," and "I tried not to talk about it." Although the scale does not specifically address avoidance in the mother-daughter bond, it is a suitable measure for assessing avoidant coping behavior (e.g., not talking about the issue). Because 2 items were mistakenly omitted, scores for the 13 items were averaged and then added twice back into the score (per instructions from Horowitz). Participants indicated their agreement on a 4-point scale ranging from 0 (*not at all*) to 5 (*often*). Thus, a higher score indicated that cancer had a stronger impact on the woman in terms of resulting psychological distress as well as more avoidant behavior. Based on their average scores, the women were placed into one of four categories, ranging from "no meaningful impact" to "severe impact event" ($N = 5$).

Relational Health: MOQ Questionnaire

The 11-item MOQ measures relational satisfaction within married heterosexual couples but has also been applied to nonmarital familial bonds (Huston, McHale, & Crouter, 1986; as modified by Vangelisti, Corbin, Lucchetti, & Sprague, 1999). The scale was modified in partner language to account for the mother-daughter relationship. Ten items are measured on 7-point semantic differentials, where participants indicate where their relationship with their mother/daughter falls along the line of dichotomous opposites. Items include "miserable-enjoyable," "hard-easy," and "free-tied down." An additional item measures relational satisfaction ranging from *completely satisfied* to *completely unsatisfied*. The mean of the sample was high at 5.97 (*SD*= .91). The measure additionally had high internal reliability ($\alpha = .93$).

Physical Health: FACT-B Scale

The FACT-B is a 36-item scale widely used in clinical trials and practice to assess the quality of life of women treated for breast cancer using four domains: social/family, emotional, functional, and physical. The 7-item subscale for physical health was used to assess the extent to which the diagnosed woman's physical well-being had been affected by her cancer and subsequent treatments. Participants indicate their agreement on a 4-point Likert scale for items including, "Because of my physical condition, I have trouble meeting the needs of my family," "I am bothered by the side effects of treatment," and "I have pain" (0 *not at all* to 4 *very much*). All items were reverse coded so that a higher score indicated better physical well-being or a low degree of impact from cancer and cancer treatments on the participant's physical health. Overall, participants indicated good physical health ($M = 3.34$, $SD = .61$), and the scale showed sufficient internal reliability ($\alpha = .81$).

Statistical Analyses

Chi-square tests of association were conducted to test SST and examine whether frequency distributions of women's social partner preferences of kin bonds differed according to a number of factors (age, disease severity, time since treatment ended). Consistent with Carstensen and colleagues' tests of SST (e.g., see Fredrickson & Carstensen, 1990), such tests of association are appropriate for assessing the relationship between categorical variables (Field, 2005). Correlations were run to assess the strength and direction of the relationship between women's mother-daughter openness communication and avoidant coping with their quality of life outcomes. Associations were tested between women's openness and/or avoidant coping, specifically mother-daughter openness (RFCP) and avoidant coping (IES), and their relational health (MOQ), psychological well-being (IES), and for diagnosed women only, their physical health (FACT-B).

PHASE 2: MOTHER-DAUGHTER NARRATIVES OF ADAPTIVE AND MALADAPTIVE COPING ACROSS THE LIFE SPAN

A multiple methods qualitative design consisting of interviews, longitudinal diaries, and diary interviews was employed to capture the quality of mother-daughter openness, avoidance, and emotional support communication as they attempted to cope together. Thirty-five dyads consisting of 78 women participated in a life-span, in-depth interview, with a subsample (N = 10) keeping a daily two-week diary and, from that sample, eight women completing a diary interview. Multiple methods were employed to allow for richer data to be collected cross-sectionally and longitudinally, capture communication during a particular disease phase (e.g., treatment), and allow for the validation of findings using triangulation.

Life-Span Interview Method

An interview was used to capture women's lived stories of their open, avoidant, and emotional support communication when coping in the mother-daughter bond as well as their perceptions of whether these behaviors enhanced their quality of life (i.e., functioned adaptively or maladaptively). The majority of women (N = 55) participated in interviews via telephone due to geographic distance. Only 23 women participated in a face-to-face interview in a research laboratory.

The individual in-depth interview was approached using a life-span method in that women described their mother-daughter communication experiences beginning before the diagnosis of cancer, across the life span of the disease, and up to the present. This made it possible to understand the changing nature of the cancer experience, the mother-daughter relationship, and communicative behavior, as well as to obtain baseline data. This also permitted assessment of women's experiences when diagnosed at different points of the life span. The individual in-depth interview protocol was semi-structured and guided by a script to ensure coverage of pertinent issues, including exploring experiences with communicative adjustment to cancer, namely, mother-daughter open communication, avoidance, and enacted support.

Modified versions of two comparable interview techniques (Lifeline Interview Method [LIM] or "flowing river of life" and Retrospective Interview Technique [RIT]) were used. The LIM is strongly recommended for life-span studies (Schroots & Birren, 2001), and RIT is also commonly used in relational communication research (Baxter, Braithwaite, & Nicholson, 1999; Baxter & Bullis, 1986; Golish, 2000; Graham, 1997). They are virtually the same method but incorporate different language (e.g., LIM embraces a sociological perspective, whereas RIT reflects a psychological and communicative perspective). Via this technique, participants receive a modified version of an RIT graph before the interview begins (see Figure 7.1). This graph provides women an opportunity to reflect on their cancer-related experience and their mother-daughter relationship.

Using the RIT graph, participants plotted turning points they experienced (both cancer related and not disease related) over the course of the disease (or its lifeline) that impacted their emotional state positively (enhanced it) or negatively (inhibited it). Time was represented on the horizontal axis, and affect/emotion was represented on the vertical axis. The upper levels on the vertical axis represented high positive affect (happy or pleasant feelings), whereas lower levels corresponded to more negative affect (upsetting, distressful, or sad feelings). On this axis, strength of mood was not specifically indicated on the graph. It was necessary to only identify the positive/negative changes in mood as a result of turning points because the primary concern was how they communicatively adjusted (using open communication, avoidance, and/or enacted support) to manage such feelings and related events.

Instructions for how to complete the graph appeared on the graph itself (see Figure 7.1). The mothers/daughters of diagnosed women received slightly different instructions in that they had to plot two lines. They plotted their perceptions of their diagnosed mothers'/daughters' lifeline of the disease in addition to their own personal experience with their mothers'/daughters' disease. This modification permitted for a better discussion of how mothers and daughters perceive they share the breast cancer transitional experience.

To obtain baseline data relating to one's mother-daughter relationship prior to the onset of cancer, each interview began with women describing their bond prior to the diagnosis. They then indicated how they felt cancer affected their relationships and whether communication changed. The interviewees also described how they communicatively adjusted (specifically with respect to open communication, avoidance, and enacted support) from the point of diagnosis to the present, their perceptions of their mothers'/daughters' behavior, and connected these behaviors with their perceived quality of life. They also described aspects of the breast cancer experience they shared with their mother/daughter, their reasons for doing so (or not), and their level of openness about their experiences. Finally, they

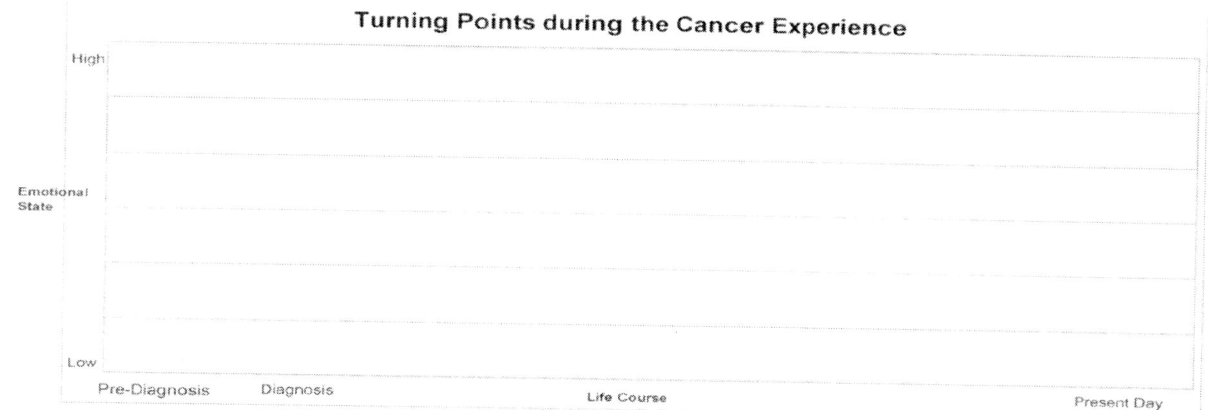

Turning Points during the Cancer Experience

INSTRUCTIONS:

There are no right or wrong answers. Everyone who completes this graph has a unique representation of their experiences with breast cancer. Please use this graph to plot out turning points you have experienced as they relate to cancer. These turning points are moments when you recall changes in your own emotional well-being. This graph is a chance for you to reflect on your experiences and take some time to recall them. We will use this graph to guide us during part of the interview.

Recall the period before you were diagnosed. Please draw a dot above the label "Pre-Diagnosis" to indicate your emotional state at that time. "Low emotional state" means you had negative feelings at that time and "High emotional state" means that you had positive emotions during that time. If you were dealing with something that was stressful (e.g., marital problems) or uplifting (e.g., recent birth of a child) in some way, please write one word or a brief phrase above the dot to note this. Next, please make a dot above the label "Diagnosis" to represent how your emotions changed once you were diagnosed.

Now I'd like you to make any dots on the graph when your mood changed positively or negatively since you were diagnosed. You may recall changes in your emotions due to a specific event (e.g., having surgery) or it may *not* be in reference to a specific event (e.g., you just recall a change in your mood for some reason). Please write a brief description of what the turning point was at that time (e.g., "ended treatment"). You may also recall turning points that didn't specifically relate to cancer but that clearly affected your mood (e.g., death of family member, new marriage in the family, etc.). You may find these important to your experience so please feel free to plot them as well. Do this up until the present day. Once you reach the end of the graph, please rate your present mood above the label "Present Day." Finally, connect the dots that you plotted with a line.

Fig. 7.1. Retrospective Interview Technique (RIT) Graph Used to Illustrate Turning Points as Mothers and Daughters Cope with Breast Cancer

shared their completed RIT graphs by discussing each turning point they plotted on the graph, how they felt at that time, how they communicatively adjusted, whether their mothers/daughters were a part of these experiences, and, if so, what specific interactions occurred.

Interviews ranged from 38 to 152 minutes long and, on average, lasted about 90 minutes. All participants gave permission to have their interviews audio-recorded. Interviews were professionally transcribed in full with a basic transcription (words spoken and notations of strong emotion such as laughter or crying), which resulted in 2,434 single-spaced transcribed pages of data. One audio file was inaudible/damaged.

Two additional means of data collection for Phase 2, the diary-interview method, were employed with a subsample of the women interviewed. The diary-interview method was primarily employed to permit triangulation with findings from the interviews. Triangulation is one way that researchers can employ multiple tools to assess the same phenomena and deepen understanding of them (Daly, 2007). Doing so enhances the validity and credibility of findings (Meetoo & Temple, 2003) and, thus, the trustworthiness of the research.

Diary-Interview Method

As previously noted, 10 women participated in the diary data collection (five dyads), with one dyad representing a case study of each age group's experiences. One dyad represented women diagnosed in young adulthood, two dyads represented women diagnosed in middle adulthood (to capture diagnosed women's experiences as both a mother and a daughter), and two dyads represented women diagnosed in later adulthood.[4] Zimmerman and Wieder's (1977) diary-interview method was employed for this method of data collection to utilize two means of data extraction. This was done via daily diary entries collected for 2 weeks followed by a personal debriefing interview. Diary entries in the study served as a means to document adaptive communication (i.e., open communication, avoidance, and enacted emotional support) in situ—in context and in the moment—over time and during a period that can be particularly challenging for families (when the patient was undergoing treatment). Only women currently undergoing treatment (either radiation or chemotherapy) and their mother/adult

[4]In the interview data, notable differences existed between diagnosed women's daughters' behavior when in their 20s compared with daughters in their 30s. Arnett (2000) distinguishes between these two age periods as emerging adulthood (ages 18–29) and young adulthood (ages 30–39). Hence, in the last age group of diagnosed women, one case study represented a diagnosed later-life mother and her young-adult daughter in her 30s, whereas the second case study represented a diagnosed later-life mother and her emerging-adult daughter in her 20s.

daughter participated in the diary-interview portion of the study. The diary was first pilot tested with three women to determine any necessary changes in procedures and materials. The pilot test also served as a verification strategy to ensure methodological congruence or coherence (i.e., that components of the method were congruent with the research question) (Morse et al., 2002).

A longitudinal design was incorporated in collecting data via the diaries. The diary-interview method as described by Zimmerman and Wieder (1977) permitted more intricate exploration of mother-daughter interactions during the challenging experience of treatment. The diary-interview method enables the collection of time-sensitive, reliable knowledge of behavior within an intensively sensitive context at a highly detailed level from the insider's perspective. Diaries are also an alternative to observation when this method is invasive (Zimmerman & Wieder, 1977). Diaries are also an ideal means for capturing individuals' communicative experiences longitudinally and as close to their occurrence as possible (Toms & Duff, 2002). By using diaries and interviews together (as is done in the diary-interview method), more detail is generated, and trustworthiness is further enhanced (Conrath, Higmethod, & McClean, 1983; Hilton, 1989; Verbrugge, 1980).

In the diaries, women were to write about their mother-daughter interactions, as well as their feelings regarding those experiences. They were also to reflect on any cancer-related thoughts they chose not to share. They recorded aspects of the interaction, such as location, length, and who initiated the conversation. Recording such features has been done in other communication-focused diary studies (e.g., see Braithwaite, McBride, & Schrodt, 2003), resulting in more descriptive results about interactions that include demographic and frequency information. The participants noted these interactive and affective experiences each day for 2 weeks. They were to make diary entries as soon after the interaction occurred but no later than bedtime. They had to keep their entries private from their mother/daughter. In line with the RIT graph or turning point approach used in the interview, mothers and daughters were also to include daily interactions that were not necessarily cancer-related. For instance, a daughter might write about an instance in which she called her mother to talk about what she did that day. These types of interactions were included in recognition of the fact that communication that is not necessarily focused on cancer is also important and may actually function in an adaptive manner. According to Duck (2008), communication scholars too often overlook the influence mundane talk can have on relationships. Thus, to capture women's communicative adjustment to cancer during treatment fully, their everyday, mundane interactions served a useful purpose.

Upon completion, participants sent their diaries to me via mail or in person. Once I received the diary, I reviewed entries to create a semi-structured interview script for obtaining more detailed information about the woman's journaled experiences. The diary interview was conducted by telephone, usually within a week of the last diary entry date. This helped to ensure women could recall detailed information about their interactive experiences. During the diary-interviews, the interviewees discussed specific entries to elucidate and amplify details concerning communicative behavior and quality of life. This procedure increased internal consistency of the entries. Some portray it as the most reliable method for obtaining diary information (e.g., Corti, 1993). As a result of time restrictions and problems reaching participants, only 8 of the 10 women keeping diaries took part in diary interviews. They ranged from 11 to 43 minutes and were 30 minutes on average. All participants gave permission to have their interviews audio-recorded. I transcribed these files. The transcriptions included only pertinent information to provide more details for certain codes and to attain saturation of categories.

Findings from the diary-interview method were presented according to Yin's (2003) single case study, embedded design. This design involves the use of a single case for several units of analysis. As such, these data were analyzed as illustrative and descriptive case studies (a case study representing each age group of dyads) and compared with the analyses of the interviews associated with the respective age group. In multiple method studies, case studies permit triangulation or comparison with data acquired via another method (in this instance, interviews) and can illustrate a phenomenon on a deeper level (Datta, 1997; Yin, 2003).

Analytical Approach

My position as researcher was to capture women's experiences in their words. Women's voices were at the foreground of analyses to bring to life their experiences. Hence, my voice and subjectivity were not relevant because I was capturing *their* stories, not ours or mine. Rather, my goal was to generate information about how women perceived their mother-daughter communicative experiences. Analysis began with interview data and was conducted concurrently with ongoing recruitment and data collection. Case studies used for the diary and diary-interview data were then analyzed and compared with the interview findings. According to Yin (2003), pattern matching involves comparing the findings from case studies with initially predicted results or, in this case, findings from the interview data. The following analytical approach was used for all of the qualitative analyses.

Glaser and Strauss's (1967) and Strauss and Corbin's (1998) grounded theory approach using a constant comparative method was employed to capture mother-daughter openness, avoidance, and emotional support in approximately 2,500 pages of interview transcripts, 141 diary entries, and an additional eight diary interviews. Grounded theory involves "the discovery of regularities" (Tesch, 1990). This approach allows researchers to examine data systematically and establish connections, and scholars can use sensitizing constructs (such as SST) to guide their explorations. The result of such analyses is conceptual ordering of the data (or a presentation of themes) to characterize mothers' and daughters' communicative experiences when adjusting to breast cancer. According to Strauss and Corbin (1998), conceptual ordering is a precursor to theorizing and "refers to the organization of data into discrete categories according to their properties and dimensions" (p. 19). Analyses were separated by age group and communication phenomena, as well as by interview versus diary and diary-interview data to allow for triangulation.

To become immersed in the data, transcripts, memos, and interview notes were constantly reviewed prior to analysis (van Manen, 1990). Data were analyzed according to van Manen's (1990) "selective approach" using the qualitative management program ATLAS.ti.6.2 (Atlas.ti Scientific Software Development, 2010). Three analytical steps outlined by Strauss and Corbin (1998) were employed, beginning with the discovery of concepts and assignment of conceptual codes to text. The analysis then proceeded with the creation of categories by grouping related concepts in an effort to reach "thematic salience." Thematic salience was reflected in recurrence, repetition, and forcefulness (Owen, 1984).[5] When possible, category labels were generated in vivo to maximize trustworthiness of the findings. The final step involved refining themes and identifying dimensions that characterized these categories to ensure thick description. According to Geertz (1973), thick description provides the domain and detail of participants' experiences—or in this case, mother-daughter communicative adjustment. In the last analytical step, the categories were reviewed again to identify similar descriptions, quotations, and ideas while making a note of these for descriptive purposes.

---

[5]Although frequency was used as a criterion of thematic salience, frequencies were not calculated for organization and presentation of themes. Code frequency is useful only for a structured interview (so all participants receive the exact same questions) and when a sample is random (see Daly, 2007). In an emergent research design, frequency of participants' responses would be directly related to the frequency of questions. Sampling relates to the kinds of experiences or specific activities to develop theory. Questions were strategic in some interviews but not in others. In other words, as thematic patterns (categories) emerged across interviews, questions were strategically implemented into future interviews as a way to build theory. Thus, frequency of codes does not provide any additional information in this design. According to Daly (2007), "Assigning numbers can be misleading. Rather, the focus needs to stay on the way the presented categories reflect the shared and patterned experiences of participants" (p. 234).

In addition to presenting thematic findings, the analyses are presented in the form of thematic action phrases and statements to increase the utility of these findings for health intervention design and implementation (Sandelowski & Leeman, 2012). Rather than only present short labels or single word codes of emergent categories in the text, the topic labels (themes) are presented as action phrases in the text presenting each typology. These are then converted into tables presenting action-oriented thematic statements that can be more easily integrated into interventions and psychosocial materials in an effort to enhance mother-daughter communication and oncology care. This approach is in line with Sandelowski and Leeman's recent recommendations for health research to be more easily translated into practice. Findings are also presented in tables using Banning's (2003) "ecological sentence synthesis" approach (see also Sandelowski & Leeman, 2012) to thematic statements.

Ensuring Trustworthiness Throughout the Multi-Method Phase

Like quantitative approaches, qualitative studies require procedures and design to ensure the research is sound or rigorous—thus, useable—or in qualitative terms trustworthy and credible. In quantitative terms, scholars must determine reliability and validity. In the 1980s, the terms *reliability*, *validity*, and *rigor* were replaced in qualitative inquiry with the concept of "trustworthiness" (Guba & Lincoln, 1981, 1982; Lincoln & Guba, 1985; Morse et al., 2002). Specifically, the research must satisfy the following criteria: credibility, transferability, dependability, and confirmability. According to leading qualitative and mixed-methods scholar Dr. Janice Morse and colleagues (2002), "Reliability and validity have been subtly replaced by criteria and standards for evaluation of the overall significance, relevance, impact, and utility of completed research" (p. 14). Hence, these criteria are useful in evaluating the trustworthiness of a study *after* it is complete rather than ensuring rigor *throughout* the research process. They further state, "Strategies to ensure rigor inherent in the research process itself were backstaged to these new criteria to the extent that, while they continue to be used, they are less likely to be valued or recognized as indices of rigor" (p. 14).

Qualitative scholars argue that indices of reliability and validity should still be used in interpretive scholarship to ensure rigor *throughout* the research process. Even though scholars in Great Britain and Europe still use the terms *reliability* and *validity* in qualitative inquiry, only a few scholars do so in North America (Morse et al., 2002). They argue that these criteria are applicable in all scholarship as "the goal of finding plausible and credible outcome explanations is central to all research" (Morse et al., 2002;

see also Hammersley, 1992; Kuzel & Engel, 2001; Yin, 1994). Morse (1999) claims that by ignoring the centrality of reliability and validity in qualitative research, scholars promote the belief that qualitative inquiry is unreliable, invalid, lacking in rigor, and, essentially, not science. According to Morse et al. (2002), the terms reliability and validity should be used in qualitative inquiry. They also argue against introducing parallel terminology and criteria because doing so can marginalize qualitative scholarship from mainstream science. They note,

> Compounding the problem of duplicate terminology is the trend to treat standards, goals, and criteria synonymously, and the criterion adopted by one qualitative researcher may be stated as a goal by another scholar. For example, Yin (1994) describes trustworthiness as a criterion to test the quality of research design, while Guba and Lincoln (1989) refer to it as a goal of the research. . . . While strategies of trustworthiness may be useful in attempting to *evaluate* rigor, they do not in themselves *ensure* rigor. While standards are useful for *evaluating* relevance and utility, they do not in themselves ensure that the research will be relevant and useful. (see http://www.ualberta.ca/~iiqm/backissues/1_2Final/html/morse.html)

Morse et al. (2002) claim that qualitative researchers should ensure the study's utility by employing verification strategies throughout the research process (instead of only after the study is complete), thereby making it a criterion to test the quality of the research design (see also Morse et al., 2002). They argue that the investigator should be responsible for the rigor of the study rather than the readers or participants (which Guba & Lincoln [1981] note can be a threat to validity). Verification includes

> Checking, confirming, making sure, and being certain. . . . [It] refers to the mechanisms used during the process of research to incrementally contribute to ensuring reliability and validity and, thus, the rigor of a study. These mechanisms are woven into every step of the inquiry to construct a solid product . . . [by] forc[ing] the researcher to correct both the direction of the analysis and the development of the study as necessary. (Morse et al., 2002, p. 9; see also Creswell, 2007; Kvale, 1989)

In line with Morse and colleagues' approach, I employed verification strategies throughout the research process to ensure that the study design and findings were rigorous. The verification strategies included attention to thinking theoretically; investigator responsiveness and flexibility as well as theoretical sampling and sampling adequacy to ensure saturation of themes; collecting and analyzing data concurrently; methodological coherence/congruence; triangulation; an active analytic stance; an audit trail including conceptual, operational, and reflexive memos; and a presentation of rich, descriptive findings.

Part IV

THE CENTRALITY OF FAMILY COMMUNICATION TO WELLNESS AFTER A CANCER DIAGNOSIS

8

THE IMPORTANCE OF FAMILY COMMUNICATION TO BREAST CANCER COPING

> *Despite widespread evidence of the profound impact of serious medical illness on family life, as well as equally compelling data concerning the role of family behavior in shaping both detection and the clinical course of medicaL illness, families are still often ignored or, at best, tolerated in many health-care settings.*
> (Baider, Cooper, & Kaplan De-Nour, 2000, p. xxiii)

To further establish that family communication should be integrated more so into cancer care and on a consistent basis, an argument that places family communication at the heart of survival and well-being is optimal. Socioemotional selectivity theory (SST) places our interactive experiences—human communication—as central to survival. As the specific prioritization of family communication in the context of breast cancer had yet to be investigated, a test to extend the theory in this manner was warranted. In addition, connections among women's quality of life, family communication, and coping behavior were investigated to further justify that family communication is central to wellness after a breast cancer diagnosis (see also Fisher, Fowler, Canzona, & Peterson, 2013; Fisher, Fowler, & Wolf in process; Fisher & Nussbaum, 2014).

PRIORITIZING FAMILY COMMUNICATION: EXTENDING SOCIOEMOTIONAL SELECTIVITY THEORY

Of the women recruited who had been diagnosed with cancer, 9 were young adult women, 18 midlife adults, and 12 later-life adults. In line with previous illness research testing SST, age would decouple from time if cancer resulted in an "ending" experience. In other words, regardless of age, one may expect that after diagnosis, women would prefer interaction with kin. Interestingly, however, these women still exhibited age differences in their communicative partner preferences, χ^2 (2, N = 39) = 7.23, $p < .05$, with a moderately strong relationship between partner preference and diagnosed women's age (V = .431). Only 44.4% of young adult women identified a family member as their first choice compared with 83.3% of women in middle adulthood and 91.7% of women in later adulthood.

Because the nature of breast cancer as an "ending" experience had yet to be tested, further analyses were conducted to better understand how cancer may fit within the SST framework. Although psycho-oncology scholarship suggests that cancer affects women's time perspective once diagnosed and makes it more limited, the unique nature of cancer as a time-centered event is unclear. Cancer is not a terminal diagnosis in the sense that not all individuals diagnosed with the disease will die of cancer. Although the diagnosis causes individuals to consider their mortality, the *extent* of this change in time perspective is not fully understood. Two disease-related factors likely affect the magnitude and length of women's time perspective change: the disease stage at diagnosis (i.e., how life threatening it is) and how long it has been since women underwent cancer treatment (i.e., how close in time to the present day is their experience with cancer).

Stage at Diagnosis

The stage at diagnosis (0–IV) of the disease is an indicator of the severity of breast cancer and, therefore, how threatening it is to one's life. As such, the disease stage likely affects women's time perspective or how life threatening the diagnosis is perceived as women diagnosed in later stages also report more stress-related symptoms (Boyer et al., 2002). The National Cancer Institute (NCI) designates "early stage" breast cancer to include stages 0–II and one type of stage III (A). A woman diagnosed in a later stage (e.g., III or IV) will likely feel that her life is more threatened compared with one diagnosed in earlier stages (0–II). Hence, it is plausible that women in later stages will have a more limited time perspective. If this were true, according to the theory, these women would likely prefer communication with kin more than women diagnosed in the earlier stages.

To explore this, women were divided into two groups: (a) those diagnosed in stages 0–II ($N = 25$), and (b) those diagnosed in stage III or IV ($N = 13$). One woman in later adulthood was excluded because she did not provide this diagnostic information. Because two categorical variables (each with two categories) were used (a 2x2 contingency table), Yates' correction was also employed to control for a Type I error (Field, 2005). The analysis suggests a connection between disease stage and family communication. A significant difference between the two groups, χ^2 (1, $N = 38$) = 6.13, $p < .05$, surfaced. A moderately strong relationship between partner preference and stage at diagnosis was found ($V = .402$).

All 13 women (100%) diagnosed in stages III or IV preferred family partners compared with only 64% of women (16 of 25) diagnosed in earlier stages. As 100% of women diagnosed in the later stages (Group 2) preferred family partners, no age differences were evident among the three age groups (four women in young adulthood, four in middle adulthood, and five in later adulthood). Regardless of age, women diagnosed in stage III or IV experienced a time perspective shift that presumably led them to prefer communication in kin bonds. Additional analyses involving age differences in Group 1 (women diagnosed in stages 0–II) (5 women in young adulthood, 14 in middle adulthood, and 6 in later adulthood) indicated that when women were diagnosed in earlier stages, age-related differences still existed in partner preferences, χ^2 (2, $N = 25$) = 11.15, $p < .01$ ($V = .668$). None of the women diagnosed in young adulthood preferred kin communication partners compared with 78.6% of women diagnosed in middle adulthood and 83.3% of women diagnosed in later adulthood. Hence, it appears that when women are diagnosed in earlier stages, their time perspective is not necessarily limited.

In light of this finding, the extension of the theoretical tenets of SST should include the stage of the disease. Women diagnosed with a more life-threatening or later stage of breast cancer (III or IV) will prioritize family communication as central to their survival.

Time Lapse Since Treatment

Another disease factor to consider is the time lapse since one's last treatment. Women continue to have regular follow-up appointments and tests for 5 years after surgery, radiation, and/or chemotherapy treatments end. However, the salience of their diagnosis and the implications it has on their perspective on how threatened their lives are likely dissipates once they transition into becoming "survivors" of the disease. These characterizations vary in health care practice. Some women have been told that they are survivors once they end treatment and have negative test results. Other women perceive they are survivors once they have their 5-year post-treatment appointment with negative test results. Hence, the time-centered nature of this factor is somewhat abstract and not well understood. Moreover, it suggests women have different interpretations of when they are "done" fighting the disease—or when their life is no longer directly threatened.

These women varied in time since last treatment. Some were currently in treatment, whereas other women's treatment had ended as many as 3 years prior to their participation in the study. It is likely that those either recently diagnosed or in treatment feel that their lives are under greater threat than those not in treatment (or women considered in remission or survivors of the disease). To explore this possibility, women were divided into three groups: (a) currently in treatment (N = 11), (b) 0 to 6 months post-treatment (N = 8), and (c) more than 6 months post-treatment (N = 20). No significant differences were in evidence: χ^2 (2, N = 39) = 1.19, p = .55. Only 70% of women 6 months post-treatment preferred kin communication partners compared with 87.5% of women 0 to 6 months post-treatment and 81.8% of women currently in treatment. In another analysis, women were divided into two groups: (a) currently in treatment (N = 11), and (b) treatment ended (N = 28). Although those women in treatment did prefer communication with kin partners slightly more (81.8%) compared with women not in treatment (75%), the statistical difference between the two groups was not significant: χ^2 (1, N = 39) = .21, p = .65.

CONNECTING MOTHER-DAUGHTER OPENNESS, AVOIDANT COPING, AND HEALTH OUTCOMES

To further the argument that family communication is central to diagnosed women's wellness and survival and to begin to narrow in on mother-daughter communication specifically, correlational analyses were run to examine whether connections exist among mother-daughter openness, avoidant coping, and their health outcomes. While no significant results emerged for the mother or daughter of diagnosed women, significant associations were found for diagnosed women. The results suggest that, in part, a relationship exists between diagnosed women's avoidant coping behavior and health and their mother-daughter openness and health.

Analyses indicate a strong positive relationship between openness in the mother-daughter bond and diagnosed women's relational health. Diagnosed women who reported a more open mother-daughter communication pattern also exhibited better relational health (r = .755). In addition, diagnosed women who reported more avoidant coping also exhibited poorer physical health. A moderate negative relationship was found in that diagnosed women who engaged in more avoidant coping also reported poorer physical health ($r = -.413$). While no relationship was found between communication or coping behavior and psychological health, this outcome may have been influenced by the missing items on the scale when the data were collected.

In summary, openness in the mother-daughter bond and avoidant coping both seem to be critical behavioral facets of diagnosed women's quality of life. These findings further suggest important links between mother-daughter coping behavior and diagnosed women's well-being.

PLACING FAMILY COMMUNICATION AS CENTRAL TO CANCER CARE

Although the test of SST did not show that women of any age diagnosed with breast cancer prioritize family communication partners, findings do suggest that this is true when women are diagnosed with more life-threatening stages (III and IV). Moreover, women in treatment may have heightened emotional needs and limited time frames (therefore, more prioritization of family communication). However, more research is needed to ascertain the complexities of this time factor in the cancer experience. Ultimately, extending SST in this manner advances our understanding that family communication is prioritized after a breast cancer diagnosis. In line with the theory, then, family behavior is central to women's ability to cope with disease and maximize well-being and survival.

With this in mind, family communication may become a preferred manner in which late-stage breast cancer patients fulfill emotional goals that are most critical to their present well-being. Analyses from the communicative behavior and quality of life data further show that the nature of that family interaction is tied to diagnosed women's health outcomes. Namely, communication in the mother-daughter bond (e.g., openness) and avoidant coping have important implications on diagnosed women's quality of life after a breast cancer diagnosis. Women with more open mother-daughter bonds also experience healthier relationships whereas those engaged in more avoidant coping tend to experience poorer physical health.

While these results are based on a rather small sample and should certainly be validated in other studies, Phase 1 of this foundational study provides theoretically driven evidence as to why kin should be considered an important component of women's quality cancer care to more fully maximize their wellness, particularly for women diagnosed in later stages of the disease and possibly those in treatment. The theoretical implications imply practical value for professionals working to improve the lives of these women and their families. These findings offer a framework that health professionals and interventionists can utilize to advocate for integrating kin interaction into care and continue to enhance or build on psychosocial resources that attend to enhancing their family communication.

Additionally, the findings suggest a tool that might prove useful in intervention work. The results using the Family Communication Patterns (RFCP) instrument help demonstrate that established open patterns of communication in mother-daughter bonds are fundamental to diagnosed women's social health. While other communication research has shown links between avoidant behavior and psychological and social health (e.g., Donovan-Kicken & Caughlin, 2010, 2011), these results show that avoidant coping behavior may also impede patients' and survivors' physical quality of life. Given this, the RFCP tool may be particularly important for identifying mothers and daughters who may need more assistance in openly communicating or families that may particularly benefit from interventions designed to facilitate and encourage open dialogue.

Part V

SECRECY AND SHARING AMONG MOTHERS AND DAUGHTERS

Exploring Openness and Avoidance

> *Actively holding back or inhibiting thoughts and feelings undermines the body's defenses . . . [and] can affect immune function, the action of the heart and vascular systems, and even the biochemical workings of the brain and nervous system . . . [placing] people at risk for both major and minor disease. . . . Not disclosing thoughts and feelings can be unhealthy. Divulging them can be healthy.*
> (Pennebaker, 1990, p. 2)

Knowing our human communicative experiences are powerful is half the battle, but refining our communication skills so that our interactive experiences have therapeutic results is a more challenging feat. To fully capture the joys and pain of mother-daughter interactions after a breast cancer diagnosis and enhance mothers' and daughters' communicative coping, we need to hear their stories. Their voices need to be prioritized in this psychosocial map of cancer coping. We need to allow the women experiencing this health crisis to teach us about their experiences in their own words, from their own perspective, using their own voice. By doing so, we extend our understanding of the role of mother-daughter communication in breast cancer coping by means of the stories of women who have been through it.

Parts V, VI, and VII illustrate the nature of mother-daughter openness, avoidance, and emotional support when coping with the illness in young, middle, and later adulthood. Special attention was directed to the context (e.g., relational dynamics and cancer-related issues) in which the participants enacted such behaviors and whether their interaction enhanced their ability to cope (i.e., the adaptive functioning of mother-daughter communication). While the analysis of these data focused on the adaptive functioning for diagnosed women, because they were also concerned with how their mother/daughter was coping, the impact of communicative behavior on the healthy partner's wellness is addressed at times in their illustrations of coping.

In Part V, each chapter represents the nature of mother-daughter openness during a particular developmental phase of diagnosis. Following are the women's authentic stories of what they shared with their mothers and daughters while coping, their reasons for doing so, as well as what they kept private or hid and why they maintained some secrecy in an effort to cope in a healthy manner. Themes are presented for each of these communicative aspects of openness for each age group of diagnosed women.

The chapters begin with a brief discussion of the developmental phase of life in which the women were diagnosed to further expand on the context of coping with an illness at various points across the life span. Contextual information about a diagnosis during that age period is also presented and based on Oktay and Walter's (1991) research, one of the only studies to date to examine the nature of breast cancer according to the age period in which women were diagnosed. This introduction is followed by demographic characteristics of the women in that age group who shared their experiences as part of my foundational study.

Across each chapter, similarities and differences in women's mother-daughter communication are discussed to highlight the unique experiences of women according to their developmental maturity. Similarities or repeated categories in typologies were included in the presentation of findings to account for subtle difference in how women describe that behavior depending on their given age group. This was done to ensure that mothers and daughters can find themselves in these stories and better relate them to their own experiences. To further visualize the similarities and differences women experience across the life span, Table 11.1 is included at the end of Part V to collectively present the typologies according to each age group.

9

DIAGNOSED IN YOUNG ADULTHOOD

Daughter-Mother Dyads

I call her right away and tell her. . . . She wants to know things right away too. If I don't call her right after I have a doctor's appointment or something, she gets worried. [She'll call and say] "Oh! How was everything? You didn't call me!"
Diagnosed Young-Adult Daughter

I think I always agreed with what she said. I never disagree or put her down. . . . I was glad that she did include me because I know some people, they think it's real private and won't discuss it. . . . I told [my children] too if something bothers you, talk about it. Don't hold it in and hold it back. I said then nothing gets fixed.
Mother of a Diagnosed Young-Adult Daughter

Young adulthood is a time in which adulthood has been reached and adolescence has ended. It is marked by a period of notable change and growth. Industrialized countries have seen a shift in the nature of young adulthood in the last few decades as more individuals pursue higher education, delay marriage and parenthood, and return to their parents' home after having moved out for the first time during adulthood. These demographic shifts have led to two distinct developmental periods after adolescence and before midlife: emerging adulthood (ages 18–29) and young adulthood (ages 30–39) (Arnett, 2000).

Young adults are still on some level cultivating their sense of self, a more defining developmental task in adolescence that often extends into emerging adulthood. In opposition to emerging adulthood, however, young adults are typically more independent by this phase of life and have established autonomous lifestyles from their parents or family of origin. While emerging adults are typically less mature, still cultivating their own worldviews separate from their parents and developing cognitive skills in decision making and problem solving, young adults are more established and comfortable on their own (Arnett, 2000). Once they have reached young adulthood or at some point during this period, they encounter life-changing developmental tasks that alter how they relate to their parents, such as getting married or establishing long-term romantic relationships and becoming a parent. For daughters, in particular, such turning points typically lead to a more understanding and egalitarian bond with their mothers (Fischer, 1986).

When women are diagnosed in their 30s or during young adulthood, they encounter a number of re-evaluations (Oktay & Walter, 1991).[1] According to Oktay and Walter's work, some described re-evaluating their professional lives or the meaning of their work whereas others re-assessed their future lives. Dealing with an uncertain future appears to be a notable challenge facing diagnosed young-adult women. Childless women expressed concerns with future childbearing, and those with children shared worries with how much to tell their children and how to take care of them when sick. Women in their 30s also described concerns with sexuality, namely, the impact of treatment on sexual desire and sensation. Some young-adult diagnosed women in Oktay and Walter's study grappled with self-blame for the diagnosis or feelings of unfairness, what the researchers called "letting go of the just world idea." Daughters' maternal bond was also impacted. While women diagnosed in their 20s easily turned to their mothers for support (or family of origin), women diagnosed in their 30s had a harder time. These women felt a tension of not being able to return to the mother-child bond (being taken care of and maybe at times wishing they could) while experiencing notable adulthood turning points (such as marrying or becoming a mother) that increased intimacy in how they related to their mothers.

[1]Oktay and Walter's (1991) research was conducted prior to Arnett's (2000) ground-breaking research distinguishing the 20s and 30s as emerging and young adulthood. Oktay and Walter sampled women in their 20s and 30s and presented their experiences collectively as women in "young adulthood." Interestingly, however, in their presentation, they separated the daughters' experiences by those in their 20s and those in their 30s as they noted a distinction in their experiences.

THE WOMEN

The following findings are based on interviews conducted with seven young-adult daughter-mother dyads and a single diagnosed daughter (N = 15). The eight diagnosed women ranged in age from 30 to 39, with an average of 34.62 (SD = 3.34). Three were married, one was engaged, and four of the women were single. Five were diagnosed with stage II breast cancer, two women had stage III cancer, and one woman was in stage IV (this woman had a recurrence). All had undergone surgery (a mastectomy), radiation, and chemotherapy. Four women were still in treatment, and the other four had some sort of treatment within the previous 18 months. Seven of their mothers participated. Their mothers varied in age from 52 to 74, with an average of 59.29 (SD = 7.45). Half the mothers were in midlife, and half were in later adulthood. Four mothers were married or remarried, one was in a long-term relationship, one was divorced, and one was a widow.

DISCLOSED TOPICS

When women were diagnosed this early in the life span, the cancer-related stressors they experienced were distinctive compared with women diagnosed later in life. These unique concerns are inherent in their disclosures to their mothers. Young-adult daughters mostly described openly talking with their mothers about the physical nature of breast cancer or procedural issues. While some women also included their mothers in their experiences with more emotional aspects of coping, this was described to a lesser degree.

Managing Treatment Side Effects

Daughters often shared with their mothers their experiences with side effects from surgery, radiation, and chemotherapy treatments. Although breast cancer treatment affects women both physically and emotionally, these daughters typically focused on the physical nature of side effects (e.g., fatigue and surgery recovery) in their disclosures. In particular, they talked openly about fatigue, appetite loss, nausea, nail disorders, and memory loss (also called "chemo fog" or "chemo brain"). They also shared their experiences with surgeries or lumpectomies and mastectomies. In these instances, the daughters talked with their mothers about their struggles with managing drains, wound cleaning, and soreness. In addition, daughters talked to their mothers about procedural issues related to side effects. For instance, daughters sometimes explained procedures they had to follow to cope with side effects. One daughter, whose career involved lifting, shared with her mother her concerns with lymphedema, a serious side effect that causes a woman's arms to swell and become numb after surgery due to lymphatic fluid build-up. To prevent this outcome, she had to rigidly restrict arm movement, which not only altered her home life but also her professional future as she had to change her job. Her mother sometimes questioned this decision:

> My mom knows I'm scared of lymphedema. . . . I just explained to her why I can't do my old job. . . . [I said] "Mom, I have this—I can get this lymphoedema thing." It was just a swelling of the arm. . . . I can get that and this is how to prevent it and that's it. (14b)

Rarely did daughters discuss with their mothers emotional effects of treatment (e.g., depression or anger). However, when daughters talked about three specific physical side effects (infertility, hair loss, or weight gain), they sometimes described the emotional nature of these challenges. For instance, some daughters opened up about what menopause was like and, thus, their experience with infertility much earlier in the life span. Although these side effects can be temporary, they can also be permanent. Most of these young-adult daughters did not have children, and some shared their concerns with their mother about whether they would be able to do so in the future. Other daughters focused these disclosures more so on the physical aspects of the side effects (e.g., exploring fertility options [harvesting eggs before treatment] or how to cope with hot flashes due to menopause).

The most common emotionally charged disclosure about side effects was when women lost their hair. Daughters often involved their mothers in their emotional preparation for hair loss. For example, daughters described engaging in activities prior to hair loss, usually before chemotherapy started, to buffer the trauma of losing their hair. Some women cut their hair extremely short or shopped for head scarves or wigs. Their mothers were often included in these monumental events. Still, many daughters described the process of losing one's hair, or how it came out in handfuls or "clumps," as very upsetting. Some openly shared these emotions with their mothers as the following daughter (who had recently had a recurrence) recalled:

> I think the most devastating thing both times was the hair loss. I mean I bawled. I was so upset. . . . I mean I had a mastectomy and reconstruction—but you can hide those things. But the hair! You know you have wigs that are good and stuff, but it is a huge, huge, HUGE part of yourself and it is devastating. I mean that's probably my lowest part, and it sounds vain but it's really, really devastating. (34b)

Mothers described sensing their daughters' emotion with this side effect, especially their feelings of loss of control in terms of how and when their hair fell out. They seemed quite aware of how emotional a loss this was for their daughters.

Additionally, daughters sometimes talked about their emotional challenges with weight gain during chemotherapy. Weight gain was a common side effect of chemotherapy as women were also taking steroids. Although most of the mothers had never been diagnosed with cancer themselves, this side effect was often easy for mothers and daughters to relate to. One mother who had not been diagnosed herself but had struggled with her weight in the past shared her daughter's emotional experience with this side effect:

> She called me yesterday and she was so excited because she lost 2 pounds. . . . It's really hard. She's very frustrated. She says, "I will not go to a certain size." But I was there [having weight gain]. I know what she's going through. It's hard—yes. (21a)

Facing Disease Risk and Prevention

Daughters and mothers also openly discussed breast cancer risk and prevention. This topic concerned screening tactics such as mammograms and genetic testing as well as understanding their family medical history of cancer. Mothers and daughters described openly talking about family history as they contemplated why the daughter was diagnosed. Oftentimes discussions involved a third party such as the diagnosed daughter's sister(s). Much of these interactions centered on understanding their disease risk and how to protect oneself and each other. One daughter expressed this concern in her discussions with her mother:

> I do tell her, "Well, you and my sister need to get checked" or whatever, in the hopes that they can prevent something. . . . She does harp on my sister like "Okay, you gotta get your mammogram done! You gotta get this done!" That drives my sister crazy, but in the same sense, she doesn't want her to go through what I went through. (34b)

Ultimately, the daughter's own diagnosis heightened the family's awareness of their own risk. Some daughters also felt that their openness about these concerns was characteristic of their lives and their communication becoming more health conscious or focused.

Some daughters described openly talking about more complex steps for minimizing future risk of recurrence or reducing a loved one's risk of developing the disease. Because these women were young when diagnosed and sometimes had a prominent family history of the disease, they often had the option of undergoing genetic testing to determine whether they carried one of the genes linked with breast cancer risk. In these instances, their mothers, daughters, and sisters also had the option of having genetic testing conducted. Not surprisingly, then, for these dyads, family history and genetic testing became a prominent focus of discussion that included contemplating the pros/cons of knowing or not knowing you carry the gene mutation. Sometimes these discussions were strictly private ones between the mother and daughter. Privacy seemed most critical when the women were waiting on genetic test results to protect younger daughters or sisters who could be affected by the outcome.

Navigating Medical Decisions

Diagnosed daughters also recalled openly discussing their medical decisions with their mothers, primarily with regard to treatment options as some had to decide whether to have chemotherapy. Others recalled having to choose to have either a lumpectomy or mastectomy. A few involved their mothers in these discussions quite intensely by talking through the benefits and costs associated with each decision and going to appointments together. However, most daughters described being open about medical decisions with their mother only after they had made the decision. As one daughter stated,

> It's more reflecting on test results. Because any decision like with my mastectomies or anything that I have done like that has pretty much been my decision and like my husband's—us talking together and stuff. I think anything I've shared with her has been just to tell "This is what I've done. This is what I'm going to do." (34b)

Daughters seemed to be open about this topic in an effort to keep their mothers "in the loop." Although sometimes daughters' mothers voiced an opinion, many seemed to understand that daughters were informing them and not asking for their insights or approval.

MOTIVATIONS FOR SHARING

Daughters described various reasons for sharing these topics in their mother-daughter bond, and at times these motives were linked to specific topics of disclosure. Their motives were clearly tied to their efforts to cope in a healthy manner or maximize their quality of life while adjusting to stresses related to breast cancer. Thus, daughters' motivations for sharing these topics were associated with how their openness could function adaptively in their adjustment as well as their mother's.

Protecting My Mother

A primary motive for disclosure by daughters was to try and buffer their mothers from unnecessary or added stress. By openly communicating, daughters perceived that they could protect their mothers from negative outcomes like the mother worrying about the daughter, the mother misunderstanding something, or the mothers being unnecessarily surprised by information because they did not hear it from the daughter first. These motives seemed to be connected to topics of openness that concerned daughters' treatment side effects as well as updates regarding medical appointments and tests.

Daughters were aware that their mothers worried about them. These daughters felt that by keeping them informed of how they were doing, they could lessen their mothers' anxiety or prevent unnecessary worry. One daughter talked about this motive in relation to updating her mother after having medical appointments:

> I call her right away and tell her. . . . She wants to know things right away too. Like if I don't call her right after I have a doctor's appointment or something, she gets worried. [Then she'll call and say] "Oh! How was everything? You didn't call me!" (34b)

To protect their mothers, daughter also sometimes kept them informed to prevent any misunderstandings or surprises. One daughter who lived in a small town and worked at the same company as her mother described how important it was that she inform her mother first before other family members or friends talked to her:

> I think that she wasn't surprised. Anything that I told her she didn't hear from anybody else, which I think would be hard for a family member if they heard it you know from a friend. . . . I think it was very important for her to know the truth all the time. (21b)

Although these motives sought to protect mothers' wellness, daughters also expressed a sense of responsibility for their mother's well-being. Thus, they acted to prevent any unnecessary distress for them. Doing so likely also enhanced daughters' own peace of mind and adjustment.

Needing Support

Daughters described being open with their mothers to attain their support as they coped with breast cancer. These women described doing so because they wanted someone there, needed advice, and/or wanted reassurance. This motive for support often coincided with wanting their mothers to join them at certain medical appointments. For instance, daughters wanted their mothers to accompany them to appointments when they were receiving test results because the outcomes could be "scary." As such, they desired their mothers' moral support. However, they also wanted their mothers' advice and reassurance at times particularly when managing treatment side effects like hair loss (insight on wigs or how to deal with hair loss) and sometimes, although less often, with medical decision making. Although most daughters told their mothers about decisions after they had made them, some reported actively involving them in their decision making. One described her motive for support with decisions:

> She was very involved. . . . I think if she wasn't there, the tendency to maybe not following through or not taking the doctor as seriously might—I don't know . . . I think I always visualize her as a person to help me make the right decisions. (22b)

A mother recalled talking through each decision by weighing the pros and cons with her daughter, as well as her husband, the daughter's father.

Still, many other daughters simply wanted their mother's reassurance about their decisions once they had been made. Mothers seemed to understand that their daughters were seeking reassurance rather than advice when they disclosed this information. As one stated,

> I think I always agreed with what she said. I never disagree or put her down. . . . She checked everything pretty thoroughly and I was glad that she did include me because I know some people, they think it's real private and won't discuss it. . . . I told [my children] too if something bothers you, talk about it. Don't hold it in and hold it back. I said, then nothing gets fixed. (34a)

When daughters' mothers recognized that their daughters only wanted to inform them of their decisions (and were not seeking advice), this motive for disclosure seemed to function adaptively as daughters were content with their mothers' responses. However, when mothers did not understand their daughters' motives for disclosure (e.g., that they wanted reassurance *not* advice), the daughters did not always perceive the interaction as helpful in their adjustment.[2]

AVOIDED TOPICS

Daughters also kept secret some cancer-related experiences from their mothers. Typically these topics were viewed by women as more "negative" in nature and centered on their uncertainty. Their descriptions of these issues also highlight the emotionally charged nature of each topic.

Grappling With an Uncertain Future

Daughters rarely shared their concerns with regard to their uncertain future. Their concerns about the future were related to fears about their mortality and disease recurrence. While women in other age groups reported this group of topics, for daughters diagnosed in young adulthood, these issues, particularly confronting death, seemed to be heightened concerns.

Daughters rarely, if ever, discussed death with their mothers. They recalled avoiding any talk about their own mortality, although many perceived it as an important and salient concern they were grappling with. At times, they struggled with the fear that they might die. They described confronting their future mortality by themselves or with another loved one rather than sharing these concerns with their mother. One daughter who had been diagnosed twice, having had a recent recurrence, shared her struggle with this:

> I've cried sometimes and broke down. Like "I can't believe I have this. I don't want to die." . . . I think that's one of those things you have to work through yourself. Like it's just one of those stages that you go through and you either, you either get through that stage, or you let the stage destroy you. (34b)

Some daughters mentioned that they may have talked about this concern with their mothers before but stressed that if they had, it was likely a rare or single occurrence. They recalled that instead they openly communicated

[2]Because this open communication is also tied to a support interaction, its adaptive functioning is examined more intricately in Part VI (see discussion of *validating decisions* in young-adult dyads' experiences).

about the issue in other relationships, such as with a husband, sister, or friend. Most mothers, too, did not recall ever discussing their daughters' mortality. The daughters' talking about death even excluded any discussion of another woman's passing. For instance, many of the daughters knew other women fighting the disease. When these friends passed away, the daughters did not share this sad news with their mothers.

Daughters with children expressed a concern about whether they would see their children grow up. One daughter saw this as a prominent emotional concern and recalled mentioning it only once to her mother but never again bringing it up. Additionally, these daughters commonly noted that they had concerns that the breast cancer would come back in the future or recur. Still, they rarely expressed this fear to their mothers. Like discussions of death/mortality, many women recalled sharing this aspect of their cancer experience in other bonds, particularly with spouses, sisters, and close friends.

Dealing With Uncomfortable or Distressing Topics

Daughters also recalled avoiding topics they characterized as negative because they were uncomfortable or upsetting. One such topic was the daughter's body image and sexuality. Many women described struggling with body image as they adjusted to changes in their breasts after receiving a mastectomy and/or reconstruction. Sometimes their concerns about body image affected feelings relating to sexuality. One daughter described this challenging adjustment in the following way:

> I don't talk too much about like the whole idea of the mastectomy and losing body parts. . . . Like now I am getting my energy back, just getting my sex drive back. I know I have like all the issues that a woman will say like, oh gosh, like fooling around with a boy and how is this going to work? But I don't really talk to [her] about that because I don't want to talk to them [parents] about my sex life. (38b)

Like other diagnosed women, this one daughter reported that instead of sharing this concern with her mother, she talked about it with female friends or men with whom she was intimate.

Another distressful topic that daughters avoided talking about with their mothers was their feelings of sadness. One recalled never sharing her emotions with her mother and only discussing medical facts associated with her experience. Daughters also avoided distressful topics that concerned their mothers' behavior. For instance, some recalled moments during treatment in which their mothers' behavior hurt them and avoided any communication about such moments with their mothers. Some never even told their mothers when they did something that upset them. Related to this topic was daughters' avoidance of their mothers' negative talk. This involved a mother's disclosures about her personal life and relative problems she was having. Daughters did not seem to want their mothers to discuss their own distressing emotional states, whether these concerns were in reference to troubles in their personal lives or about the daughters' cancer. In essence, daughters seemed to want to eliminate negatively framed discussions. Mothers often admitted avoiding such topics as well. One daughter recalled trying to avoid subjects of this nature in her conversations with her mother:

> Some subjects you just don't bring up. I don't like bringing up subjects when she's first talking about things that she thinks are wrong like just in her life or something. I think it's annoying. I'd rather say "How's the weather today? This is what the kids are doing and here's what my doctor said to me." And be done with it. Where she likes to dwell on certain things and it's like, oh my goodness! (34b)

MOTIVATIONS FOR SECRECY AND AVOIDANCE

Daughters' motives for avoiding some topics were somewhat related to their reasons for disclosure. Namely, daughters were motivated to keep some issues secret in order to protect their mothers. Yet at the same time, this avoidance was also motivated by a need to protect oneself. This motivation was linked to daughters striving to enhance their coping, which they perceived necessitated avoiding negative topics.

Protecting Myself and My Mother

As noted, some of the topics about which daughters avoided talking were ones they perceived as distressful. As one daughter stated, "I think it helps me be stronger when I don't see someone else breaking down in front of me" (34b). Another daughter reflected on how her mother often involved her in her personal problems and leaned on her for support, which was also characteristic of her mother before her diagnosis. This daughter recalled being distressed by her mother and father's behavior: "Why did they not recognize that this is big? I have a lot going on and I can't exactly take care of everything, the way they want me to" (33b).

Daughters also avoided topics to protect themselves from their mothers' reactions, which they believed most likely would be negative. For example, one daughter learned that her mother was telling her friends and family details about her experience—details the daughter had disclosed to her mother in confidence. The daughter saw her mother's email correspondence with other women in which they were discussing her experience. She felt her privacy had been invaded without her permission. In response, she avoided further discussions to protect herself from this outcome:

> She was sharing my thoughts and feelings and everything with basically everyone she knew. . . . That is a problem! . . . They were talking about me and I just wasn't happy with that. . . . [Now] I just give her the [medical] facts. I will never talk about my feelings. (33b)

Some daughters also recalled censoring what they shared with their mothers to buffer them from unnecessary distress or worry, the same reason they also disclosed some aspects of their cancer experience. Oftentimes they avoided showing their concerns about their uncertain future, as when waiting for test results. For example, one daughter shared her experience about recently finding another lump. She admitted that she had not shared this with her mother. She stated,

> I didn't tell her that . . . I didn't want to worry people unless—in case it had been nothing. . . . I'll deal with it if I have to deal with it. . . . There's not necessarily anything to deal with right now. So it was a wait and see kind of thing. (15b)

This example of daughters' avoidant communication was similar to how they sometimes delayed telling their mothers about their diagnoses. Many recalled waiting to tell their mothers that something was wrong until after the lump had been biopsied and had a definitive diagnosis.

Daughters also kept secret their fear of recurrence to prevent their mothers from experiencing distress. Many daughters were adamant about avoiding this topic of talk. As one daughter stated, "No. God no! No one knows about that. . . . There's no point in putting out stress to my mom. Knowing that I'm worried! No, no, no, no. Why worry her? No way" (14b). Many women avoided discussions about their own mortality for this reason as well. One daughter talked about how this topic of talk would only cause her mother and father distress:

> I don't want to upset them. . . . I don't think breast cancer is going to kill me, but if it does, I decided that would be okay too. . . . I haven't informed them with that because they would not be fine with that. I think that will just be too much for them to think about or to bear. . . . But once I realized that, it was almost like this huge weight was lifted. I feel free like it doesn't make me sad or anything. I just felt good. (38b)

10

DAUGHTERS AND MOTHERS DIAGNOSED IN MIDLIFE

I know [my daughters] really don't want to talk about it. I mean, it's too much to deal with it right now—worrying about breast cancer and them getting it. . . . Every now and then if I have an opportunity I'll say something, but they probably don't like it . . . It is really hard when you're a mother . . . you do want to talk to your children about it.
Midlife Diagnosed Mother

I didn't really know how to react to it so I kind of hid from it and I kind of blocked it out of my mind . . . just looking at her and knowing that she might not be there next year killed me. . . . I shut everybody out at first. And I was just like I'm in my box and you're not going to come in.
Daughter of a Diagnosed Midlife Mother

Health issues—I was pretty open with her about things like that. You know, it's like nothing tastes right and I don't have an appetite or I'm starving.
Midlife Diagnosed Daughter

She had several trips to prepare for the reconstruction. . . . She's very open about it and I was too. I appreciate the fact that she was close to me in that regard.
Mother of a Diagnosed Midlife Daughter

Midlife, one of the most overlooked phases of development in aging research, has been rightfully framed as a "juggling act" (Fingerman, Nussbaum, & Birditt, 2004). During midlife, women have familial ties with generations above or older than them (e.g., parents, grandparents), below them (e.g., children or grandchildren), and with their own generation (e.g., spouse, sibling, cousin). Not surprisingly, then, this is the only chapter that includes diagnosed women's openness and avoidance experiences in both roles or as a daughter and a mother. A midlife adult's social network is often at its most expansive as women juggle more roles (parent—provider—spouse—adult child or caregiver—professional—friend). Midlife can be a time in which they are pulled in multiple directions at once, oftentimes at the expense of their own individual needs. While women in midlife vary in their experiences given individual differences in life and familial experiences (e.g., presence or age of children, grandparenting roles, career status and demands, marital status, economic status, and family origin ties), middle-aged adults share three developmental goals that are at the core of their communicative experiences (Fingerman et al., 2004). Midlife is a time in which responsibilities increase, namely, associated with the management of multiple, sometimes conflicting roles one encounters during this period (Erikson, 1963). While identity development is still a core element of young adulthood, this task continues in midlife, becoming more complex, which may include for some women a new identity shift (La Sorsa & Fodor, 1990). This may be particularly true for divorced women who re-enter the world of dating, become single parents, or become part of a blended family. Last, women in middle adulthood are more aware of a less time expansive future and, at the same time, conscious of consistencies from their past (Neugarten, 1968).

When diagnosed in middle adulthood, the women in Oktay and Walter's (1991) study described struggles with individual needs and redefining bonds. Individual challenges included identity renegotiation as women refocused on their body image, femininity, and self-reliance. Many women felt an urge to help other women coping with the disease, which may be tied to their new developmental need for generativity, a developmental task of giving back. Midlife women also described relational challenges in their marriages and with children. Some recalled husbands not commonly voicing concerns or that the women did not directly express their needs. Those with adolescent children expressed struggles managing their child's developmental need for separation and that teenaged daughters, in particular, seemed to exhibit problems. Some recalled their children as sources of support, which may be linked with their friendships changing, including, for some, a withdrawal from their friends. While some women also recalled midlife as a time in which their mothers depended more on them, breast cancer was an opportunity for moms to support daughters.

Some diagnosed women described this as particularly important whereas others did not experience a supportive relationship with their mothers.

DAUGHTERS DIAGNOSED IN MIDLIFE

The following findings derived from interviews with five middle-adulthood daughter-mother dyads and two single diagnosed daughters (N = 12). These seven diagnosed women ranged in age from 42 to 51 and had an average age of 46.00 (SD = 3.00). Six were married, and one daughter was in a long-term relationship. Five were in stage 0 or I, one was in stage II, and one daughter was in stage IV (this woman had a recurrence). All seven women had undergone surgery (lumpectomy or mastectomy), two also had radiation therapy, and two women had undergone chemotherapy. Only one was still in treatment at the time of the interview. Four had received treatment within the previous 12 months and two daughters within the previous 24 months. Five of the daughters' mothers participated. Mothers ranged in age from 65 to 83 and averaged 72.60 (SD = 6.58). All of their mothers were in later adulthood. Four were married, and one was a widow.

DISCLOSED TOPICS

Daughters diagnosed in midlife had a different experience of openness with their mothers compared with all of the other mothers and daughters diagnosed at other points during the life span. Like daughters diagnosed in young adulthood, the topics they chose to share were predominately physical in nature. However, their disclosures did not include emotional experiences and were much more pragmatic in nature.

Managing Treatment Side Effects

Daughters in midlife openly and frequently shared with their later-life mothers their physical experiences concerning side effects from cancer treatments. These conversations tended to be more casual than serious in tone and typically consisted of daughters explaining and complaining about various side effects, including loss of appetite, change in taste buds, breaking out in rashes, hot flashes from chemotherapy-induced menopause, headaches, problems with digestion, nausea, and vomiting. Some described their disclosures as similar to telling their mothers how they felt when they were sick or ill (in a non-cancer-related scenario). These daughters recalled keeping the discussions factually or medically focused. For example, one daughter explained that she openly discussed only "health issues" (i.e., side effects) with her mother:

> Health issues—I was pretty open with her about things like that. You know, it's like nothing tastes right and I don't have an appetite or I'm starving. And I want to eat this and this is something I usually can't stand. That kind of thing was weird. (24b)

Daughters' disclosures concerning side effects seemed to help mothers determine when to call their daughters. One mother noted how the open communication would work for her. She referred to side effects in a similar fashion (physically focused) to the daughters:

> She was pretty open about how it [chemotherapy] affected her and how she felt about it and that was usually, you know, when you've got a headache and you don't want to move your head. You sure don't want to talk to anybody. And so I would wait until she felt like talking, or she would call me when she finally felt better. (10a)

As a result, these disclosures seemed to function adaptively for both mothers and daughters by keeping mothers abreast of her daughter's experiences but also cuing them as to when would not be a good time to talk or connect.

Staying Informed About Diagnostic Testing and Results

Daughters also shared their diagnostic tests and results with their mothers. Some openly talked and offered this information voluntarily whereas other women recalled only sharing if their mothers asked them to. As in the case of side effects, the daughters frequently mentioned being careful to supply only factual information related to medical updates. As one daughter stated, "I didn't give her a whole lot of information" (35b). Although daughters shared only factual information and did not go into details, their mothers seemed to appreciate their daughters keeping them informed about their medical appointments and experiences. Doing so helped the mothers understand how their daughters were doing. Many mothers mentioned keeping calendars of their daughters' appointments. One indicated this in relation to her daughter's reconstruction appointments: "She had several trips to prepare for the reconstruction. . . . She's very open about it, and I was too. I appreciate the fact that she was close to me in that regard" (24a). Daughters seemed to be at ease in disclosing this information with their mothers so long as it remained factual or medical in nature.

Navigating Medical Decisions

Midlife daughters spoke openly with their mothers about the medical decisions they made. Such decisions included whether to have a mastectomy, reconstruction choices, and treatment options (e.g., radiation and/or chemotherapy). However, these were not necessarily interactive. In other words, unlike some young-adult daughters, midlife daughters never involved their mothers in the decision-making process and provided information about medical decisions after they had already made the decision alone or with some other loved one. As one daughter explained, "I didn't say, 'What do you think of that?' I might have said, 'Do you have any questions?' Or something like that. . . . My husband and I really made that decision up front" (11b). Likewise, mothers recognized that these were personal decisions for their daughter, and possibly daughters' husbands, to make. Interestingly, mothers sometimes admitted that they purposely did not offer their opinions. They most often described this behavior in reference to daughters' decision to have a mastectomy. Mothers often indicated they felt the daughter should make the decision herself.

Only one daughter recalled her mother interjecting an opinion after she had openly talked to her about a decision she had made. She indicated how her mother's response led her to no longer openly share her decisions:

> I told her that I was doing research and I was talking to people too and I said I think that based on what I am finding out, I am going go ahead and do, you know, what I feel is best. And I just listened to what she said but I didn't tell her I was not going to listen to it. . . . I had already made my decision. . . . She would talk to somebody she knew and she got back to me and she said, "You should not have that" and "You should not have radiation." But, you know, that is how she reacts and that's why I didn't discuss it with her because she couldn't just objectively talk about the information. She just got emotional right away. (35b)

MOTIVATIONS FOR SHARING

Unlike daughters in young adulthood, midlife daughters rarely offered reasons for their openness. Rather, they merely reinforced that, in order to cope in a way that maximized their own health, they consciously stuck to medical or factual topics. They perceived that straying from pragmatic aspects of the breast cancer experience (i.e., or talking about anything emotional in nature) would only inhibit their ability to cope.

Sticking to the Facts

The previously reviewed topics that daughters openly discussed with their mothers indicated that they only disclosed factual and medical aspects of their cancer experience. When directly asked what they shared with their mothers, daughters often responded by saying they disclosed only factual information. Reasons for this restriction varied. A few interviewees felt that their mothers did not fully understand the cancer process. Because of this, they explained that it was best to keep any conversations about their cancer strictly factual. One daughter noted, "I was sort of the one educating her" (5b). Some daughters explained that because their mothers wanted to "keep track" of the appointments or procedures, it was easier to focus on medical or factual information. Finally, other daughters felt it was too traumatic for their mothers to talk about anything cancer-related except for the physical aspects as one daughter observed:

> I think it was hard for her too. I think she didn't absorb it. It was like, it was almost like she was [the one] hearing that cancer diagnosis. You know how you—the patient—right away doesn't hear it? I think that was what happened to her. I don't think she really heard what I was saying the first few times I talked to her about it. (35b)

For daughters, then, by openly communicating only about physical aspects of breast cancer or the facts, they minimized distress for both themselves and their mothers. Hence, this motivation is somewhat tied to a desire to protect their mothers as well as themselves from emotional distress.

It is also noteworthy that all of the daughters' mothers were in later adulthood, a generation that tends to be more closed in terms of emotional expression, and most of the daughters were in early, less life-threatening stages of the disease (0–I). Not surprisingly, then, most of their experiences with treatment were significantly less than those diagnosed in young adulthood. Many only had a surgery for treatment, an experience that may be more medically focused and less emotionally charged than care plans that also involve radiation and chemotherapy.

AVOIDED TOPICS

Both mothers and daughters frequently described not being consciously avoidant with respect to cancer-related issues. Rather they felt that they just did not talk about certain topics. As a result, daughters and mothers provided little information about specific avoidant behavior. Although diagnosed daughters did not frequently mention open communication with their mothers about many different cancer-related topics (e.g., hair loss, emotional side effects, body image), the only topic they admitted avoiding, albeit somewhat indirectly, was with regard to their future.

Grappling With an Uncertain Future

Although a few women admitted that they once talked to their mothers about issues related to future uncertainty, they described it as a rare occurrence. More commonly, women did not discuss this. Cancer-related topics that were characterized as future uncertainty included mortality or death and seeing one's children grow up.

However, diagnosed daughters did discuss these topics with other loved ones, namely, their husbands or friends. They mentioned they did not feel that they consciously avoided these topics with their mothers possibly because most were diagnosed in early stages, and, thus, their experience with breast cancer was not as life threatening compared with many of the women diagnosed in other age groups.

MOTIVATIONS FOR SECRECY AND AVOIDANCE

Daughters diagnosed in midlife also did not readily provide reasons for avoidant behavior. This is not entirely surprising as they also did not feel they actively avoided cancer-related topics. Yet in reviewing their discussions of what topics they openly talked about or avoided (however indirectly), two inter-related reasons emerged that are suggestive of daughters' motivation for avoidant behavior.

Protecting My Mother

Some women mentioned their concern that disclosing to their mothers would only cause them more worry. One woman tied her concern to her mother's age and struggles with anxiety. Another woman referred to being apprehensive to talk openly about her cancer for fear she would upset her mother by "laying" too much on her: "Sometimes you do not want to lay that much on, you know what I mean?" (7a). Daughters' mothers were in later adulthood with an average age of 70 years. Moreover, the mothers often did not live geographically close by.

Talking to Others

Although diagnosed women in this age group did not feel they actively avoided topics, they admitted to talking about certain topics only with their husbands, sisters, and/or girlfriends. Sometimes women felt that those were just issues about which they could more easily share with these particular loved ones. In addition, it seemed that these daughters could interact in more depth about certain issues with other individuals than their mothers.

MOTHERS DIAGNOSED IN MIDLIFE

The following findings relate to interviews with 12 middle-adulthood mother-daughter dyads (two dyads had two daughters participate) and one single diagnosed mother (*N* = 27). Only 12 of the 13 diagnosed women returned information about their background, although some of this information emerged in their interviews. Diagnosed women ranged in age from 44 to 52, with an average age of 49.42 (*SD* = 2.50). Ten were married, one was in a long-term relationship, and one was divorced. Most women were in stage 0 or I breast cancer (*N* = 8), two women were in stage II, and three mothers had stage IV cancer. Two of these women had experienced a recurrence. Of the 10 women who reported full treatment histories, all had undergone surgery (mastectomy), 7 also had radiation therapy, and 6 also had chemotherapy. Three women were still in treatment, three had undergone treatment within the past 6 months, four had within the past 24 months, and one within the prior 36 months. Fourteen of these mothers' daughters participated. The daughters ranged in age from 18 to 29 and had an average age of 20.64 (*SD* = 2.90). All were emerging adults. Nine were single, and five were engaged or in a long-term relationship. Many of them still lived with their mothers at the time of diagnosis, as well as during treatment.

DISCLOSED TOPICS

Mothers' communication with their daughters was often factually based, much as was the case of the other middle adulthood dyads' experiences and daughters diagnosed in young adulthood. However, these diagnosed women had a separate and unique experience in their role as mother. These mothers seemed to agonize more about which cancer-related topics to share with their daughters because they were concerned about their daughters' vulnerability. Hence, although mothers may have discussed some cancer-related issues with their daughters, they typically did not go into detail.

Their daughters were also aware of this aspect of their interactions. Moreover, the mothers often admitted that because their daughters lived with them at the time of their diagnosis and/or during treatment, their daughters were unavoidably exposed to their cancer experience. As such, although the topic of cancer talk was similar to other mother-daughter pairs, the dynamics of their interactions were quite different.

Managing Treatment Side Effects and Procedures

As with the previous age groups, mothers often shared with their daughters their experiences relating to treatment, namely, their recovery from surgery and struggle with side effects, as well as treatment procedures. Both mothers and daughters recalled that these discussions focused mostly on what mothers underwent physically, as well as the logistics or mechanics of the treatment procedures (or what was involved). Unlike the other age groups of dyads, mothers' disclosures were more educational in nature.

The mothers talked openly with their daughters about their side effect experiences with fatigue, hot flashes, and hunger cravings, but they tended to only disclose "basic things" or the physical aspects. They also admitted that they rarely gave their daughters details. One described her openness with her daughters in this manner:

> What they do know is that I have horrible heat flashes now and that type of thing so they do know about that part of it. But I'm not sure if they know how much of a big deal they think that is. I tend to downplay medical type things. (26a)

Mothers often seemed to disclose such information to their daughters to help them better understand what was happening to them, but they kept details related to feelings to themselves.

The mothers also talked about and showed their daughters their surgical scars throughout the healing process. One recalled using the *Show Me* book (a well-known publication displaying women's mastectomies) so that her daughters could look at other women's bodies in case they were uncomfortable looking at hers. Mothers explained sharing the physical aspects when they felt it would help their daughters better understand their experiences. Sometimes their daughters were interested in seeing the physical changes, but not all wanted to discuss or visualize their mothers' surgical experience. Interestingly, this difference in comfort level was often notable when the mothers had two daughters with distinct personalities living at home. One daughter described how seeing her mother's scars helped her understand the bodily changes she had to endure and felt this openness helped her withdraw less from her mother. She also compared it to her sister's experience:

> My sister doesn't deal with blood. . . . She would probably pass out. . . . I saw every aspect of her side effects and it was not too fun. She had drainage pipes on the side and the fact that those were constantly pulling and it's like—no, it's not right. Something shouldn't be coming out of your body from inside like that—[It] has to hurt. So it's seeing that and realizing how much pain she actually is in made me realize, all right, I guess I got to be a little bit more receptive to this than I am. (16b)

The mothers also shared with their daughters the logistics and procedures involved with treatment. At times, they did so over the telephone to daughters who were away at school. In other instances, they brought their daughters with them to radiation or chemotherapy treatment. This was not a common occurrence, as most daughters were in school, and the mothers had their treatment during the day. However, many mothers recalled bringing their daughters to treatment at least once so they could see what the visits involved. Mothers seemed to be attempting to minimize any fears their daughter had. As one stated in relation to her chemotherapy appointments, "I was just trying to take the scariness out of it for them" (16a). The mothers and daughters often indicated that such openness did have that effect. One noted that by being open, her daughters would have a role model in case they ever had to face the disease in the future. Unlike the other dyads, mothers' openness seemed to relate to educating their daughters about the experience to minimize fears they may have had.

Facing Daughters' Future Disease Risk and Prevention

Daughters' prevention was also a common topic. Mothers and daughters talked freely about genetic testing, mammograms, and family history. Unlike young-adult diagnosed daughter-mother dyads, this openness centered on how daughters of diagnosed moms must proactively protect themselves from developing the disease. Sometimes the discussions arose after daughters expressed to their mothers their concerns about developing the disease. However, mothers admitted that more often they had to initiate these talks. They indicated that they wanted their daughters to understand that breast cancer was an important matter about which they should be concerned, but they did so in a manner that would not alarm them unnecessarily. For instance, mothers often reassured their daughters that their chances of developing the disease were not high. As one said:

> I want her to be concerned with that. I do want her to be sure she starts getting checked early and that kind of thing. . . . Telling her that as long as she does the proper things and being checked and that type of thing, it's very treatable now. (26a)

Although the mothers often discussed daughters' prevention efforts, both noted that this was not a major concern to them because they perceived their daughters were young. Still, most mothers brought up the topic at least once and stressed the importance of talking about prevention. The mothers tended to initiate these conversations periodically throughout the cancer experience. The daughters recalled these talks occurring once in a while, which seemed to make sense to them in light of their age. At times the discussions coincided with mothers showing their daughters their surgical incisions so that daughters could see what happened to them during treatment.

Daughters varied in their responses to their mothers' openness about their future disease risk. Many daughters seemed to be uneasy discussing this matter at times. They tended to withdraw and, if possible, avoid this topic—behavior that is further explained in the subsequent presentation of avoidance in this bond. Some daughters seemed to want their mothers to talk about such matters. Doing so appeared to be particularly important to the mothers' well-being in knowing their daughters would be careful in the future. For instance, one mother recalled talking to her daughter the day of her diagnosis about her own prevention and asked her to have a "workup" as soon as possible. The mother recalled her daughter's response: "I want to." Additionally, daughters sometimes talked about wanting to engage in prevention immediately. At times they even noted being upset when their doctors refused to give them a mammogram until they were at least age 35.

Interestingly, these daughters sometimes admitted they felt guilty about being concerned with themselves. One observed that she felt reassured but guilty at the same time:

> She told me like I better always go get mammograms and she didn't go. She skipped a year and the lump could probably have been caught earlier. So she said she'd never do that again and that I should go. But she's also said that most people's breast cancer isn't hereditary. . . . It made me feel a little bit better but then it made me feel bad that I was worried about myself getting it when she actually had it. (26b)

Mothers also described feeling guilty but for different reasons. They experienced guilt because their daughters had to consider that cancer might be part of their future, something they regarded as unfair because their daughters' lives were just beginning. Possibly related to this, some mothers mentioned their doctors' telling them not to "burden" their daughters with this topic yet.

MOTIVATIONS FOR SHARING

Some daughters were living at home with their mothers because they were still in high school at the time of diagnosis or were home for a summer or holiday vacation from college. Living together influenced how much mothers talked about cancer with their daughters. Mothers often noted that it was impossible for their daughters not to know certain things (or for certain things not to be discussed) because they lived at home. This did not appear to be a reason for openness but rather an indication as to why daughters were exposed to certain things. Instead, mothers seemed driven to disclose by one particular factor: their daughters.

Sharing Because My Daughter Wants Me To

Whether daughters wanted to know seemed to have the greatest influence on what cancer topics mothers decided to openly talk about. This motivation directly related to the daughters' comfort level with their mothers' diagnosis versus desire for information concerning how the mothers were doing (as was the case with the other age groups of dyads). Mothers often mentioned being open only as much as their daughters wanted them to be or when their daughters wanted to know things. As one mother of several daughters put it, "I'm open with them if they want the information. It's there. It's not that they want it exactly" (20a). Many mothers noted wanting to be open with their daughters. However, they felt that their level of openness or what issues they were open about depended on their daughters' wanting to know about those experiences. These mothers seemed to understand that their daughters had varying comfort levels in hearing details. The mothers also indicated that their daughters' comfort level was important because of their young age. Because of this, they recognized that their daughters did not always want to talk about certain matters. They also noticed that for cancer to surface in a discussion, they often had to initiate the subject.

The daughters' desire to know varied. Some women recalled daughters wanting to know "everything" and always asking, "What's next?" These daughters tended to ask their mothers questions often. One mother recalled her daughter saying, "Well, the more information I have will certainly help me in the future when I make my own decisions" (27a). In opposition, other women recalled daughters not wanting to talk about cancer, sometimes ever. In these cases, there was often more than one daughter in the family, one of whom was comfortable with the subject and the other not.

Yet the educational nature of mothers' openness also seemed inherent in their motive for disclosing when the daughter wanted information. At times mothers felt it was important for their daughters to acquire information. They integrated these topics during interactions in which they thought the information would be more easily received. For instance, mothers talked more openly about cancer when the topic had already been raised (e.g., they were talking about a friend's diagnosis, something came up on television, or the mother had a doctor's appointment). Although the mothers seemed to understand that their daughters' maturity affected how open they could be, avoidant behavior from their daughters sometimes was difficult to negotiate.[1]

AVOIDED TOPICS

These mothers' avoidant experiences were similar to middle-adult diagnosed daughters' in that avoidance was described in relation to issues not coming up versus actual conscious avoidance. Mothers and daughters indicated that certain topics did not come up—sometimes because they felt it was not something they had thought about (e.g., death/mortality), other times because they were too busy, and still others because it never surfaced in any conversation. However, they often explicitly stated that they did not perceive that if a topic did not come up or was not mentioned, this meant they were avoiding the issue. Rather, they perceived that the topic did not seem applicable to their experiences with cancer. Mothers only frequently mentioned actively avoiding talk about one particular cancer-related topic, and daughters also seemed to be aware that their mothers avoided this subject.

Hiding Negative Emotions

Many mothers indicated that they kept their emotional distress to themselves. Some women recalled experiencing negative affect related to side effects (e.g., their feelings were more sensitive), as well as their emotional concerns about cancer in general. They described actively hiding any distressful feelings from their daughters. As one mother stated, "I tried not to get really upset. . . . I have to turn my emotions on and off" (30a). In turn, daughters also recognized that their mothers avoided this topic. When asked whether her mother shared any emotional distress, one daughter stat-

---

[1]This avoidant communicative experience was a notable aspect of mother-daughter communication in this group of dyads. Hence, it is discussed further in this group's experiences with avoidant behavior as well as enacted emotional support (see talking versus withdrawing) in Part VI.

ed, "I think she was experiencing stuff like that, but she never really talked about it with me." Some daughters said they knew their mothers shared those feelings with other people (e.g., a close friend).

Although mothers talked about consciously avoiding this subject in discussions with their daughter, at times it was unavoidable because the daughters were still living at home. One mother described this type of situation. This woman recalled not being able to control her emotions all the time because the treatment and medications minimized her ability to do so. Because both her daughters lived at home, they were often together:

> I think I would have kept that [sad emotions] internal. I don't think I would talk to either of them about it. Although what seemed to happen for me was like I would cry very easily about things. That was very obvious to them because out of nowhere, they would be kidding or whatever, and I seemed ultra-sensitive to things. . . . I felt like I could cry at the drop of a pin and I was very sensitive. . . . They obviously noticed and they probably felt like they had to walk around things a lot and be more cautious because there were frequent episodes where I would just cry. (26a)

Although daughters were aware of the emotional nature of their mothers' experience, they rarely discussed it or sought to determine how their mothers were feeling. It was a topic that they consistently tip-toed around.

MOTIVATIONS FOR SECRECY AND AVOIDANCE

Mothers' reasons for avoidance had to do with their daughters' well-being. Many mothers avoided this type of talk to prioritize their daughters' wellness. As noted, most daughters were just out of high school, and diagnosed women seemed more concerned about how their daughters were handling the diagnosis. As such, they discussed two reasons for avoiding this talk to prioritize their daughters' wellness.

Responding to a Daughter's Withdrawal

Both mothers and daughters mentioned many cases when daughters did not want to talk about anything cancer-related. For some mothers and daughters, this characterized their relationship throughout the cancer experience. Although mothers worried about their daughters' withdrawal, they seemed to feel their daughters' avoidant behavior was sometimes helpful to their well-being and adjustment. This was also important to mothers who tended to worry about how their daughters were coping. One mother explained how she made sense of her daughter's withdrawal behavior, saying, "It is a way to protect your mind from too much heavy stuff" (20a). Daughters often did not want to hear about their mothers' treatment side effects, medical decisions, or concerns regarding genetics and their need to take preventive steps to avoid developing the disease. Daughters reportedly showed avoidance by changing the subject, ignoring their mother, making jokes, staying away from their mothers, leaving the house, going to their rooms, or blatantly telling their mothers they did not want to talk about it. In response to their daughters' withdrawal, mothers avoided cancer-related talk.

Mothers interpreted daughters' avoidance in different ways. For instance, they sometimes felt that their daughters were too young and not ready to deal with certain cancer-related topics. In these instances, they portrayed the daughters as ignoring the topic or making light of it. One mother reflected on her daughter's avoidance in this way when she tried to talk to her about genetics and prevention. This mother had tested positive for a breast cancer gene mutation and had additional surgery (oophorectomy) to minimize her risk of recurrence. As a result, she was especially worried about her daughters' potential for developing the disease. Her daughters, who were in their early 20s, did not want to talk about this issue. The mother recalled:

> I know they really don't want to talk about it. I mean, it's too much to deal with it right now. It's overwhelming to think about—worrying about breast cancer and them getting it. . . . Every now and then if I have an opportunity I'll say something but they probably don't like it that I say something. . . . It is really hard when you're a mother, though, because you do want to talk to your children about it, but when they don't want to talk about it and then so you really have to—it's a fine line of not being obsessed with it. . . . You would like them to come to you or something or just so they come to terms with it. . . . I think I would bring it up if it came [up]. I wouldn't bring it up myself. I think I would bring it up if we were doing something together or we found out somebody else got breast cancer or something like that that would bring up the topic. . . . They wanted to ignore it for now. I think that's fine. . . . [Referring to one daughter] She'll deal with it when she needs to deal with it. (20a)

The mothers often felt that their daughters avoided cancer talk because they were protecting themselves. Their daughters presumably were upset about the diagnosis, and avoidance was their way of coping. Because of this, these mothers often believed it was necessary to mirror their daughters' avoidant behavior.

The daughters also often described their avoidant behavior in ways that appeared to validate their mothers' experiences in that it was a means of protecting themselves. As one daughter stated, "If you have to talk about it, it makes it more real, so avoiding it kind of made it less real" (26b). One daughter, who was a senior in high school when her mother was diagnosed, described such an experience:

> I didn't really know how to react to it so I kind of hid from it and I kind of blocked it out of my mind . . . just like looking at her and knowing that she might not be there next year like killed me. . . . I was angry about it but I don't think that's why I pulled away. I pulled away 'cause that's like the only thing I knew that I could do to help myself through it because I'd be a mental wreck. . . . It was easier for me at the time just to shut it out of my mind and just pretend nothing was happening. . . . Once she stared chemo it hit me that like, hey! I got to accept this or else it's just going to keep haunting me for this entire thing. So I finally did. . . . I shut everybody out at first. And I was just like I'm in my box and you're not going to come in. (16b)

This daughter eventually talked more openly after going to a therapist. A few other mothers also had their daughters see a therapist or counselor to help them stop avoiding the subject and start talking.

Some mothers recalled avoiding topics because their daughters had always been uncomfortable or queasy about medical subjects. Daughters often found this avoidance as natural for them, in that they could not stand the thought of anything medical (e.g., blood or surgery). Their mothers also talked about the avoidance as consistent with their daughters' comfort level with physical or health issues. However, most mothers mentioned their daughters not wanting to talk about cancer in relation to the stress it caused. Avoiding or withdrawing was the daughters' way of minimizing their own distress.

Although the mothers seemed to understand that this avoidance was what their daughters sometimes needed, the daughters often felt guilty about their behavior once their mothers entered recovery or survivorship. As one daughter observed, "Looking back, I probably could have been a little more focused on her and asked more questions about how she was doing and things. But just selfishly, I don't know. Maybe I thought I couldn't handle the answers" (36b). These daughters recalled how difficult it was for them to see their mothers vulnerable, weak, and upset. Still, daughters often felt the avoidance was helpful and necessary. As one daughter stated, "It is kind of better that she did not tell me some of the stuff because it was hard for me. . . . It would have made it worse."

Protecting My Daughter

Relatedly, mothers also avoided topics because they wanted to prevent their daughters from feeling distressed. These mothers did not avoid talk because their daughters withdrew but because they knew it would upset their daughters. They avoided talk about cancer to keep their daughters from worrying about them. Many made reference to the difficulty in avoiding talk in relation to the daughter's needs and well-being, as one mother in discussing withholding information from her daughters about her diagnostic tests said:

> I would hope that I was open with them, and yet, by the same token, I don't think I went overboard explaining things. Maybe I didn't give them enough information, but I tended to just gloss over things. I did not want them worrying about it. . . . I just wouldn't say anything because I didn't want them to be concerned. . . . I didn't tell them much because they were already going through enough and they were both going back to school. . . . I didn't want them worrying about me. So I didn't add all that other stuff to them. I just kind of didn't want them to see that emotionally. (26a)

Many mothers noted avoiding cancer discussions because they felt it would only distress their daughters and distract them from their own lives. Many of these mothers' daughters were starting or returning to college and involved in extracurricular activities. One mother reported feeling this way:

> I really didn't want to tell her anything. I figured she had enough to adjust to going away to school and being in [sports]. You know I think she had plenty to deal with to get adjusted to. And I wouldn't be selfish hurting her with all that until I needed to tell her. (29a)

Some mothers noticed that their daughters were initially worried after a disclosure and, hence, avoided talk in the future. As one mother said:

> She had a bad time with it. So now I'm not too honest with her unless I'm sure. . . . If it's serious then I'll tell her. In the beginning I tried to tell everything. Now I think it's too much for her emotionally. (30a)

Mothers were aware that their avoidance did not always please their daughters, even if they were trying to protect them. For instance, one mother recalled keeping information from her daughter that she eventually found out about. This mother became quite ill after her first chemotherapy treatment and had to be hospitalized. She and her husband did not call to tell their daughter because she was away at college. They did not want to disrupt her studies. When they finally told her (after the mother was home from the hospital), their daughter was furious and even responded by withdrawing from her mother communicatively. Similarly, another mother recalled not telling a daughter who was studying abroad about her diagnosis until she returned home. This daughter was also angry at being kept in the dark. These daughters recognized that their mothers did not disclose to protect them. However, they felt that they could often tell when their mother hid things and that not knowing what was wrong caused them worry. As one daughter noted:

> She does not want to make me feel bad about it or something like that. I do not know if that makes sense. . . . It would kind of bother me a little bit that she did [that], but I think she did it because she would try and hide it. And sometimes she could, but sometimes she was not good at it. (30b)

The young women in this cohort indicated that they did not always want to know or even talk about their mother's experiences related to cancer. Notable, however, is that the daughters always wanted to know when something serious had happened (e.g., mother being hospitalized) while not necessarily wanting to hear all the details of their mother's experiences (e.g., side effects) or talk about cancer topics all the time. This struggle for both mother and daughter as to what to disclose and avoid or what one wanted to hear or not hear created a difficult balancing act that they needed to constantly manage.

11

DIAGNOSED IN LATER LIFE

Mother-Daughter Dyads

I don't want everybody to know how I feel.
You know sometimes you want to hide your emotions. . . .
I don't always want to tell what I'm thinking.
[My daughter] doesn't need to know everything.
Sometimes she thinks she should.
Diagnosed Later-Life Mother

I wanted to know everything. I wanted to know all the details, and she had been reluctant to tell me. . . . I thanked her for protecting me, but I said that's not the way I want to do this. I want to hear about everything. . . . I wanted to do this as a peer and as an adult and not to have it be like she was my mom and trying to protect me. I think that would have been way scarier for me.
Daughter of a Diagnosed Later–Life Mother

Advancements in medicine have led to a longer life span, leading to extended familial bonds between children and parents and grandchildren and grandparents. Later adulthood has a hallmark of changes often characterized as gains and losses. On a relational level, women in later adulthood are typically faced with a decreasing social network and a heightened concern for emotional well-being or present wellness. They may be coping with difficult transitions such as retirement, widowhood, singlehood, remarriage, or becoming a custodial parent to grandchildren (Nussbaum et al., 2000). However, becoming a grandparent may be an especially special time in later life as women engage in mentoring, socializing, and surrogate parenting for grandchildren. On a health-related level, later life is also sometimes accompanied by mental and physical losses such as cognition, hearing, or mobility that might challenge aging women to gain new competencies to accommodate such changes. In addition, they may be managing multiple chronic conditions (e.g., high blood pressure, diabetes) in the midst of encountering challenging diagnoses. As such, these changes may impede on women's sense of independence.

According to Oktay and Walter's (1991) research, coping with loss is already a theme inherent in later-life-diagnosed women's personal lives and, as such, can be rather overwhelming after a diagnosis. Likewise, they found that women diagnosed in this age period struggled more with depression and despair compared with women diagnosed earlier in life. Some women encounter role reversals with their adult children due to health or cognitive changes that may impede their ability to make medical decisions. At the same time, this can be a time in which they seek the support of their adult children. Relatedly, the threat to one's sense of independence is an important issue for later-life-diagnosed women as they may need help but also want to maintain their autonomy. In their mother-daughter bond, then, this challenge was particularly important, and many women described a point of renegotiation as they struggled with issues of power and dependence.

THE WOMEN

The following findings related to interviews with 11 later adulthood mother-daughter dyads (one dyad had two daughters) and one single diagnosed mother ($N = 24$). The 12 diagnosed women ranged in age from 57 to 69 and averaged 61.92 ($SD = 4.48$). Eight were married, two separated or divorced, one divorced/remarried, and one a widow. Only seven knew the stage of the disease: three women were diagnosed with stage I, three in stage II, and one at stage III. All had undergone surgery (lumpectomy or mastectomy), nine also had radiation, and seven underwent chemotherapy. Three mothers were in treatment at the time of the interview. Six had some sort of treatment within the previous 12 months, two within 18 months, and two mothers had treatment within the last 36 months. Eleven mothers' daughters participated, but one did not provide demographic information. The daughters ranged in age from 21 to 51, with an average age of 31.10 ($SD =$

8.85), thus spanning three developmental periods (emerging, young, and middle adulthood). The bulk of daughters, however, were young adults (30–40 age range), and only one woman was in middle adulthood (age 51). Four daughters were married, one divorced/remarried, three in a long-term relationship, and two daughters single.

DISCLOSED TOPICS

As true of the other age groups, women diagnosed in later adulthood shared some cancer-related experiences with their daughters. Compared with the other mother-daughter dyads, however, these mothers were not typically forthcoming with information. Rather, these women often did not initially provide their daughters with extensive details about these topics. Yet because their daughters were inquisitive, they typically responded by opening up more with their daughters, oftentimes about the same topics as mothers and daughters in earlier phases of the life span. As such, while some of the shared topics are similar across the other age groups, the nature of the disclosure is somewhat distinct.

Managing Treatment Side Effects and Procedures

Later-life mothers openly discussed with their daughters their experiences with cancer treatment. Their disclosures consisted of sharing general information about what treatments they were receiving, as well as any side effects they encountered from radiation, chemotherapy, and surgery. At times mothers volunteered the information. Often, however, the daughters expressed a desire for the information, after which the mothers then began to share.

When mothers discussed cancer-related issues, they tended to share physical or medical aspects of treatment primarily. Hence, like those in other dyads, these mothers did not typically communicate about any emotionally related aspects of treatment. Some recalled updating their daughters concerning treatments they would be undergoing. Often these interactions focused on the logistics of mothers' treatment experiences, particularly when they stopped or started a new treatment regimen. One mother reported telling her daughters how she went to her radiation treatments during the week:

> I didn't really describe anything or go into a lot of details. I told them I had to go every day, five days a week at 9:30 I had to be there. It took me longer to drive to the hospital than to get treatment! You know, that was kind of a joke, like I got to be there by 9:30 but I'll be back by

> 10! It was really quick unless you had to wait for some reason. I never gave them a lot of details. Maybe after the first time and that was it. (23a)

The mothers in this age group also noted how they disclosed to their daughters their experiences with side effects associated with these treatments. Again, their openness typically related only to factual information. Side effects that mothers talked about included memory loss from chemotherapy, breast tenderness from radiation, leg cramps, stomach upset or nausea from medications, headaches, reddening of skin from radiation, fatigue, mouth ulcers, and constipation. Many mothers recalled describing their "yucky" or "creepy" days to their daughters, but they did not give their daughters many details about the side effects; instead, they restricted their accounts to physical changes or challenges they were encountering. Some even mentioned that they would not openly talk about their treatment experiences unless their daughters asked.

Mothers also sometimes shared with their daughters emotional aspects relating to mood swings from chemotherapy. Although this side effect is often associated with emotional changes, their disclosures tended to concentrate on the medical effect from treatment rather than the emotional challenges of dealing with this side effect. The daughters confirmed that their mothers' openness regarding any treatment was medically focused. Yet they also seemed to be aware that their mothers were struggling emotionally. One daughter who knew her mother had severe bouts of depression during chemotherapy (because her father told her) reflected on her mother's selective disclosures:

> [My mother] was like, "Well, it seems like the first day or after chemo, I feel this way and I don't like to eat very much" or "These are the things I like to eat. On the second day, I feel this way." Especially with the first part of chemo. Like I said, she left out the depression or at least didn't explain it to the full extent but was always like, "Here's how it goes." (9b)

Another daughter reported a similar experience:

> It was never emotional. It was always very, if I could say "clinical." It was all about the treatment. It was all about the drugs. It was about prognosis and never, never intimate [like] "How does it feel to me. . . ." (23b)

Although the mothers admitted they did not share much about the emotional aspects of the disease, their daughters often mentioned being concerned about their mothers' mental health. At times the daughters learned about their mothers' sadness or depression from other loved ones (e.g., fathers or grandmothers). Still, many times daughters were able to sense their mothers' sadness when talking over the telephone and in person. It is noteworthy that although this topic was not one that diagnosed mothers openly discussed, their daughters frequently talked about it in their interviews. Because the mothers were of an older generation, they may have been less apt to freely express their emotions. Nonetheless, it was often a pressing concern for their daughters.

Encountering Diagnostic Testing and Results

The mothers recalled that what they shared about diagnostic tests was factual in nature and related to such matters as PET scans, bone scans, MRIs, genetic testing, biopsies, and mammograms. They also reported talk about what the procedures involved and what the tests entailed, as well as what the results of tests meant. For instance, one mother noted:

> When they said they wanted to do the biopsy . . . I was on the phone with [my daughter] and just let [her] know that they wanted the biopsy. I said [to her], "Actually I've been reading on this and only 8 percent of the time does the calcification [on the mammogram] mean anything." (42a)

When the mothers shared information about procedures and talked about the results of the tests with their daughters, they often did so in conjunction with discussions of treatments.

Some women recalled keeping daughters "updated on all the reports and what they meant and what it means for them" (42a). Some daughters recalled their mothers being detailed in their explanations of test results. As one observed:

> She's very detailed. You know, my mom took notes on everything so she wanted to talk about it . . . she still needs to. She talks about it. . . . She told me word for word everything that happens, and I just listen. (19b)

Some mothers recognized that daughters wanted specifics concerning the test results, at times more so than the mother did. As one mother stated, "[My daughter] wants to know about . . . my tests, how my tests come out, because I still have a lot of tests. I guess they are more specific now—they want specifics, more details now" (12a). As with communication about treatments, sometimes mothers initiated this discussion. Other times they shared information only after their daughters asked them to.

Facing the Daughters' Disease Risk and Prevention

Mothers frequently communicated about prevention for their daughters. The women told their daughters about discussions with their physicians about daughters' future risk and actions they needed to take to minimize their potential for developing the disease. Most of the daughters were in their 20s and 30s. When the daughters were closer to age 40, discussions seemed to be more frequent compared with women with daughters who were still in college. Mothers recalled talking to their daughters about getting mammograms, doing self-exams, and becoming more health conscious. Like midlife mothers, some later-adult mothers felt their daughters did not appreciate their openness about this topic. One mother described such an interaction with her daughter who was in her early 40s:

> I said to her, "Have you scheduled your mammogram yet?" [And she says] "No, I haven't done it yet, Mom." And I'll say to her, "Well, you've got to do that. You're supposed to do that now." And then she'll say, "Well, you know, so and so down the street just had a mastectomy and she went for her mammogram the week before or two weeks before and nothing showed up, and she does the self breast examination, and she found the lump herself." So her attitude is like, which is really kind of dumb, she'll say something like, "So, you know, look at that!" And I'll say to her, "Do you do self breast examinations?" No! No she doesn't! But that's the way she is. . . . I don't know why. I just don't understand that, especially in this day and age and with my condition. (17a)

In contrast, some mothers stated that their daughters were interested in prevention. They openly communicated about this topic more easily and felt their daughters wanted to know how this disease could affect them at their age. Some mothers felt it important not to "preach" and instead to "drop a hint." One mother described how she openly communicated her concerns about prevention to her daughter in this way:

> Because they are younger, they may think they don't have to go there [medical appointments] that often, but I don't bring it up very often though. I might bring it up after I've had one, then just, kind of it's on my head, you know. [So I say] "I had mine last week. Have you got

your appointment?" And that's it. That's all I do. That usually is enough. (23a)

Daughters seemed to realize that their mothers' openness about prevention was an effort to protect them from developing the disease. Some admitted being resistant to or scared of having a mammogram. One daughter in her early 30s described this fear, saying,

> I'm worried I'm going to have it. I don't think I do. I'd probably be able to tell but I just—I'm going to do it. I'm going to do it. That's just something I've been trying not to do. I know I have to. It's like one of those things that you know you're going to do it and you know you have to, but you really don't want to. I will though. (32b)

Other daughters did not hesitate to see their doctors after their mothers talked to them about prevention. As one recalled:

> I don't even know if it would've been necessary for Mom to even tell us that we would have to do that because we knew we would have to do that now. I think it made her feel better knowing that we were going to do that. (17b)

This group of dyads' experiences was similar to those of midlife mother-daughter dyads. However, daughters of mothers diagnosed in later adulthood seemed to understand that by taking preventive steps, they helped ease their mothers' mind. Hence, these daughters realized that being open to talking about their own prevention was helpful to their mothers' adjustments to their own conditions. Although these daughters were also young, the majority were about 10 years older than the midlife-diagnosed mothers' daughters (who were emerging adults or in their 20s). This age difference likely affected comfort levels as well as understanding the significance of their mothers' openness regarding this topic.

MOTIVATIONS FOR SHARING

Like those diagnosed in midlife, later-life mothers consistently mentioned that their daughters motivated their disclosures. Yet unlike the daughters of midlife mothers, these daughters typically always wanted that information.

Sharing Because My Daughter Wants Me To

Many of the mothers stated that they were open with their daughters only because their daughters wanted to know what they were experiencing. Some indicated that they were open because they somehow just knew their daughters wanted to know. Other mothers knew their daughters wanted them to disclose and share their experiences because they explicitly expressed this. One mother recalled, "Like she said to me, she didn't want me to hide my feelings no matter what I was feeling" (4a). Daughters recalled having similar interactions. One described how her mother censored information early on. The daughter's maternal grandmother would then disclose to her what her mother was experiencing. This daughter recalled addressing this with her mother: "I said something like, 'Mom, you have to tell me how you feel. Like I want to know. I want to help you.' And she's like, 'I know but I don't want you to worry'" (32b). As this daughter pointed out, daughters seemed to want to know this information to have a better sense of how their mothers were doing.

Some mothers felt that if they did not openly communicate with their daughters, they would be upset, as one said: "I know that if they were not fully informed, they would be very upset with me for not telling them" (19a). Other women felt their daughters would be worried if they were not open, as the following mother explained:

> I just assumed [they] would want to know. And [they] did want to know. I mean I didn't have to worry that they would want to know. It was just understood that there would be—it was significant enough. I think they might have been concerned if I weren't sharing information. (42a)

Daughters also often adamantly stated that they wanted to know "everything." They felt that by knowing what was going on, they could help their mothers adjust better. Daughters also expressed that *not* knowing would be even more worrisome. Knowing everything seemed particularly important to daughters who could not be with their mothers physically because they lived far away. One daughter in her 20s, who was also a single child, described wanting her mother to be open for this reason:

> If I could really picture everything and really know exactly the process and exactly what she was going through, it helps make it more real for me but in a good way. I remember really feeling the change from when it was just this big nebulous scary thing to okay. This is how it's being dealt with. These are the treatments. These are the steps. It was able to make it more specific for me, especially because I wasn't there. . . .

> Making it as specific made it more comfortable. It didn't make it this big, giant, scary thing. . . . I wanted to know everything. I wanted to know all the details and she had been reluctant to tell me. . . . I thanked her for protecting me but I said that's not the way I want to do this. I want to hear about everything. I want to know it all. I want to know the specifics. I think that probably set the course. It did set the course for how the whole thing was going to go. She knew at that point I wanted to do this as a peer and as an adult and not to have it be like she was my mom and trying to protect me. I think that would have been way scarier for me. That was a big time. (9b)

Like their daughters, mothers often perceived that being more open helped them adjust better. Many of these women felt that it enhanced their relationship with their daughter in a new way, making it more intimate. As one mother stated, "I was glad [she wanted to know]. I wanted that to happen" (4a).

AVOIDED TOPICS

Mothers avoided talking with their daughters about two cancer-related topics. Similar to the other age groups of mothers and daughters, emotionally charged topics were withheld, although for these diagnosed women, negative affect was especially challenging compared with women diagnosed earlier in the life span.

Grappling With an Uncertain Future

Mothers admitted that they rarely, if ever, talked to their daughters about their future-oriented cancer concerns. These topics included mortality/death, survival rates, recurrence, and struggles with uncertainty about their own health in the future. Some mothers felt it necessary to bring up their potential death just once because, as one stated, "We don't know what's up tomorrow" (19a). Several admitted to being scared about death but did not discuss their fears. As one mother indicated, "No, I haven't shared that with very many. I don't want to share it with them [her children]. You know that's one thing I don't think [my daughter] and I have really said is about death" (4a).

Daughters recognized that this topic was absent from their interactions. One recalled her parents in a sense banning it from their communication: "Pretty much immediately, either my mother or father or both of them said, 'Nobody's talking about dying.' I'm sure [this was] one of the first things my mom said after she told me about being diagnosed" (9b).

Daughters also seemed to understand that even though it was not discussed, survival remained a concern for their mothers. One daughter recalled the topic coming up once but never again.

> I know the kinds of things she is thinking about and the kinds of things that make her upset or depressed through this whole thing. Questioning how long she's going to live. I know that kind of stuff stresses her out and that type of stress for my mom stresses me out. . . . We haven't really talked about that directly. Before radiation we addressed it minimally. . . . I know it's on her mind but we haven't really talked about it all. (41b)

Some mothers felt death was unnecessary to talk about because they did not believe they were dying. These women sometimes referred to the high survival rate with breast cancer. Other times they noted that mentally they were just not "there" in their experience with the disease. Hence, like midlife-diagnosed women, these mothers often clarified their avoidance in relation to the nature of their cancer experience. Yet they also admitted talking about it once and then never bringing it up again, in contrast to the earlier diagnosed age group of mothers with younger daughters, whose members did not discuss the topic at all.

Mothers and daughters also recalled that they rarely talked about recurrence or uncertainty about the future. Most mothers were open in the interview about their fear of recurrence but admitted they did not share that worry with their daughters. Daughters seemed to recognize that their mothers lived with these concerns, even after treatment. One recalled sensing these concerns each time her mother went for follow-up appointments:

> I know that she worries about [recurrence], but she doesn't bring it up much. I think when she goes for her exams, you know, we're all worried. And then, you know, her tests. But when she comes home she's like, "I'm okay." And we're like, "Oh good. We're all coming over." (17b)

Like their mothers, the daughters also avoided bringing up this topic. Many daughters reported that they let their mothers raise issues because they did not want them to feel uncomfortable or to have to think about cancer if they did not want to.

Hiding Negative Emotions

Mothers also rarely disclosed to their daughters any negative emotions they had throughout their cancer experience. They confessed to trying to hide their emotions from their daughters. As one stated, "All the negative feelings that I have, I tried to keep personal" (19a). This avoidance was noteworthy in how women talked about their side-effect experiences.

Although their mothers were not forthcoming about their emotional distress, daughters were keenly aware of their mothers' emotional states. Moreover, they realized that their mothers particularly avoided any talk about feelings of depression. Depression or feelings of extreme sadness are a notable challenge that many women encounter due to hormone changes from chemotherapy, as well as the psychological trauma of the diagnosis. Still, mothers rarely talked about the challenges posed by emotions in their mother-daughter bond. Even when mothers did share their feelings, daughters typically described them as glossing over the issue. One daughter described her mother as avoiding a full disclosure of her feelings in the following:

> She would say, "Oh I'm not feeling good today" or "I'm kind of down." But [my dad] was the one that said [to me], "These days a week, after she's had chemo, she's depressed. Seriously depressed." And made sure that I understood that it was not just like "Oh, I don't feel very well." . . . He made sure I really understood what she was dealing with. (9b)

Daughters also reported that they could sometimes sense their mothers' depression in their tone over the telephone or visually see it in their expression. Other times, daughters learned of their mothers' struggles with depression from another family member (e.g., fathers or grandmothers). Yet like their mothers, daughters avoided talking about negative emotional states with their mothers. This avoidant behavior may be associated with an understanding (on the part of both mother and daughter) that older generations are less comfortable freely expressing their emotional feelings due to their experiences growing up in a more closed sociocultural environment.

MOTIVATIONS FOR AVOIDANCE AND SECRECY

Mothers had two strong motives for avoiding cancer-related talk with their daughters. In line with other mother-daughter dyads across the life span, their reasons for secrecy were tied to the desire to buffer or protect their daughters. Yet a new, not yet described motivation also characterized these mothers' avoidant communication with daughters in that these mothers especially valued their privacy. For these mothers and daughters, an interesting tug of war for sharing the experience ensued. Daughters' desire for information (a motivation for mothers to disclose) often competed against and, at times, infringed on the mothers' need for privacy.

Maintaining My Privacy

Many mothers indicated that their reason for not openly talking with their daughters about certain cancer-related issues was to maintain their privacy. Numerous mothers explained that they were "very private people." Some felt that because they valued their privacy, they preferred to talk about issues such as death and future uncertainty with their husbands, not their daughters. As one mother observed, "Being a private person, I would've preferred not to have to do that unless it was necessary" (19a). Mothers admitted not telling their daughters "everything" because they felt they would then lose any sense of privacy. This motive seemed to be the reason mothers did not disclose to their daughters their negative emotions. One mother explained this by saying:

> I don't want everybody to know how I feel. You know sometimes you want to hide your emotions. Sometimes like I say—if I'm too down, you know, if I'm down I don't want to [answer] "What's wrong?" I don't always want to tell what I'm thinking. . . . You know maybe I have an ache or pain somewhere that I'm concerned about. . . . But I don't always tell them that so—She doesn't need to know everything. Sometimes she thinks she should. (4a)

Daughters often recognized that their mothers valued their privacy even though most daughters discussed this in relation to their mothers' behavior with hair loss. Often the daughters attempted to talk to their mothers about not wearing their wigs and instead wearing a pretty scarf or even nothing once their hair started growing back. As one daughter said, "She would never go in public without her wig on. . . . She was always covered" (19b). Mothers sometimes admitted avoiding these talks as their daughters did not understand that the wig was also a means of maintaining privacy. One mother explained, "A scarf around my head still tells people I have cancer. My wig does not. [My daughters] finally just stopped saying anything 'cause they knew I was not going to change my mind" (41a).

For mothers diagnosed in later adulthood, maintaining some privacy was important. They were guarded in terms of how much of their cancer experience they wanted to expose, and maintaining privacy also seemed to enable them more control over their disease experience.

Protecting My Daughter

Many mothers in this cohort recalled avoiding talk about cancer because they did not want their daughters to worry or be upset. In addition, by avoiding talk, mothers felt they were not making a "big deal out of it." This effect seemed to be particularly important in making sure their daughters were not overly upset by their mothers' diagnosis. Mothers had this concern because they also knew their diagnosis was, on some level, upsetting to the daughter. They seemed to believe that by not talking about anything cancer-related, their daughters would worry less.

Sometimes avoidant behavior involved censoring information, and at other times mothers delayed sharing with their daughters. For instance, some mothers recalled waiting to disclose bad news (e.g., positive biopsy results) because they did not want to ruin their daughters' day. One mother described her avoidant behavior for this reason: "Somehow I thought [the news] would change how [her day went.] . . . I really felt like well, I am going to wait about telling news like that. . . . I was thinking about protecting her, but how silly is that?" (9a). Daughters were also aware their mothers shielded them from information to prevent their becoming emotionally distraught or, as one daughter put it, a "mental case." One daughter who struggled with severe anxiety talked about understanding why her mother displayed avoidance: "I really think she was more concerned about my emotional [state.] . . . I think she was more concerned about not upsetting me at all" (42b). One mother even confessed to avoiding cancer-related talk because she felt responsible for negatively altering her two daughters' lives because of her diagnosis. She discussed her reasoning for her avoidant communication:

> All three of our lives are drastically changed from a year ago. And I hate that. And so the less I can [talk about it]—bad enough that we're doing appointments and surgeries and all other kinds of things. So I don't do it when it's not absolutely necessary. (41a)

Like those in the other age groups of diagnosed women, these mothers felt a sense of responsibility to buffer their daughters from additional, unnecessary distress. However, unlike emerging adult daughters of mothers diagnosed in midlife, these daughters, many of whom were young adults, did want their mothers to share openly with them. For these daughters, not knowing what their mothers were going through was even more distressful.

Table 11.1. Mothers' and Daughters' Openness and Avoidance

To effectively cope in this type of mother-daughter bond	*diagnosed women share these topics*	*for these reasons*	*and avoid these topics*	*for these reasons*
young-adulthood diagnosed daughter-mother bonds	treatment side effects disease risk & prevention medical decisions	protect mother seek support	future uncertainty uncomfortable or distressful topics	protect mother & self
middle-adulthood diagnosed daughter-mother bonds	treatment side effects diagnostic testing & results medical decisions	stick to factual information	future uncertainty	protect mother talk to others
middle-adulthood diagnosed mother-daughter bonds	treatment side effects & procedures daughters' disease risk & prevention	daughter wants to know	negative affect	daughter does not want to talk about it protect daughter
later–adulthood diagnosed mother-daughter bonds	treatment side effects & procedures diagnostic testing & results daughters' disease risk & prevention	daughter wants to know	future uncertainty negative affect	maintain privacy protect daughter

Part VI

COPING SIDE BY SIDE

Adaptive and Maladaptive Emotional Support

> *Understanding how social support is adapted to coping needs is also important if we wish to assist would-be support providers in offering support more successfully. . . . Simply advising someone to offer . . . nurturant support gives little guidance as to the form, content, style or sequence that might be most effective.* (Goldsmith, 2004, p. 114)

Part V offers a deeper understanding of what aspects of the breast cancer experience diagnosed women share with their mothers and daughters as well as what they tend to keep secret, private, or avoid talking about. In analyzing their open and avoidant behavior, a clearer picture emerged of the nature of how mothers and daughters share many aspects of coping with the disease. In examining their motives or reasons for doing so, it is possible to also ascertain how and why mothers and daughters are open or avoidant and how those communicative behaviors are engaged in an effort to cope in ways that maximize each other's wellness in the face of a life-threatening illness.

To extend this further, it is important to examine how mothers and daughters support one another while sharing these cancer-related experiences. To understand diagnosed women's experiences of enacted support from their mothers/daughters, both the women's and their mothers/daughters' interviews were analyzed. Numerous types of behaviors surfaced. Some enacted support communication was perceived as helpful and, thus, always adaptive in diagnosed women's adjustment to their condition. Other supportive communication ostensibly functioned both adaptively and maladaptively, meaning the same forms of support sometimes helped women cope and at other times was perceived as unhelpful or unhealthy. Context appeared to be what best accounted for this variability. In other words, contextual factors like the breast cancer-related issue at hand or the mother or daughter's age mattered. Like the previous analysis, analyses of emotional support were centered on the adaptive potential of behavior for diagnosed women. However, as was noted in women's openness and avoidance interactions, diagnosed women were also quite concerned with how their mother/daughter was faring, and, as such, this impacted their behavior. Thus, the influence of support behavior on their partner's wellness is also sometimes noted in their narratives.

In Part VI, each chapter represents the nature of mother-daughter emotional support communication during a particular developmental phase of diagnosis. Emotional communicative support behavior that appeared consistently to function adaptively and enhanced mother-daughter coping is the initial focus. This is followed by emotional support that was sometimes helpful in disease adjustment and in other instances unhelpful. Mothers and daughters' narratives highlight how and why support functioned in these conflicting ways. As was done in Part V, similarities and differences in women's mother-daughter communication are discussed across the chapters to capture the distinct nature of emotional support at various points in the life span and ensure that families who read this book are better able to relate to and transport themselves into these mothers' and daughters' lived stories. Table 14.1 is presented at the end of Chapter 14 to provide typologies of emotional support across each age group of mother-daughter dyads.

12

COPING IN YOUNG ADULTHOOD

Daughter–Mother Dyads

I like it in that she will offer "Whatever you need. Just tell me." But not you know—not pushy about it. Not "Oh I want to come down there. I'm coming down. I'm taking care of you!" . . . She sort of left it up to me and I liked that. I was sort of like "Okay, I actually need you to come down now." . . . She was really happy when I asked. She wanted to be wanted that way and didn't want to impose that on me and ask.
Diagnosed Young-Adult Daughter

I'd just check in periodically. . . . I have to remember, too, that she's not feeling well this day [treatment days]. . . . I'd phone a couple of days later to give her a chance to recoup a little bit and then see how things were. Or, you know, I'd phone [daughter's husband]. . . . I kept thinking, you know, when you're sick, the last thing you want is 50 million people phoning you to see how you're doing, even if it is your mother.
Mother of a Diagnosed Young-Adult Daughter

As was evident in young-adult daughters' accounts of openness and avoidance, it was important for these diagnosed women to be the ones to set the tone for how they would share the breast cancer journey with their mothers. At the same time, some of these daughters were without a significant partner and without children, which made issues such as companionship and concern for the future more urgent. Their reflections depict the importance of negotiating support in the mother-daughter bond in this phase of a diagnosed woman's life span and the potential for a mutually beneficial experience of coping together.

ADAPTIVE ENACTED EMOTIONAL SUPPORT

Four types of enacted support communication were recurrently described by women as consistently functioning in an adaptive manner in that this mother-daughter communication enhanced their ability to cope and adjust to stressors encountered while navigating breast cancer. The women illustrated how support was enacted to manage specific issues associated with the disease and, therefore, had an impact on their well-being, as well as how their behavior was a means of negotiating this shared experience. The interconnected nature of daughters' openness and avoidance with emotional support communication are also at times described in their accounts of coping together.

Being Willing to Listen

Daughters felt that when their mothers carefully listened to them, it enhanced their disease adjustment. Listening was especially important when daughters shared their emotional feelings and concerns with their mothers, which was not a common disclosure for daughters. In these instances, daughters admitted that they wanted their mothers simply to listen, to let them talk, often without any input. One daughter described her need for this type of support: "Sometimes you just like to vent. . . . She's always willing to listen" (34b). When mothers listened, daughters felt they had the opportunity to vent, express their concerns, and cope with cancer in their own way. One daughter expressed how her mother enacted this type of emotional support: "She doesn't correct me or tell me how I feel" (22b).

Mothers seemed to understand that, at times, their daughters needed them just to listen. Hence, they remained silent and allowed their daughters to deal with their concerns as they needed. For instance, one mother stated, "I just listen. . . . She has to deal with it the way she has to deal with it. So I don't like to put in my two cents" (22a).

Showing Affection

Showing affection always helped daughters in their adjustment to cancer. Several daughters recalled receiving affection from their mothers more frequently soon after the diagnosis. Most often they received more hugs from their mother. Mothers also recalled saying "I love you" frequently. At times, this form of enacted support represented an effort to provide comfort to the daughters. Such affection was especially comforting for daughters who experienced hair loss due to chemotherapy treatment. One reflected on how upset she was when her hair fell out in clumps quite quickly. She recalled, "I came out of the shower crying and she put her arms around me. . . . [She was] taking me in her arms and letting me cry because it was a shock" (13b). In addition, mothers showed affection to comfort their daughters when they received upsetting information. For instance, some recalled moments when their daughters were emotionally upset and sometimes cried after receiving disappointing test results from their physicians. During such times, mothers noted how they consoled their daughters sometimes silently but with a warm embrace.

Being Humorous

Daughters indicated that humor was especially helpful in coping with their cancer experience. One daughter noted that humor "kept us on air." Often humor centered on treatment side effects or outcomes, specifically changes in the daughter's body. For example, women joked about hair loss, mastectomies, plastic surgery, and menopause. Their humorous behavior ranged from jokes to teasing. One dyad even went to laughter therapy together. All of the daughters in this cohort felt that telling jokes, teasing, and laughing together made the atmosphere more comfortable and, hence, the adjustment to cancer easier.

A common way of enacting this support was for mothers and daughters to create humorous nicknames. These nicknames typically referred to bodily changes after treatment. For instance, women adopted various nicknames to characterize their hair loss. These names included Uncle Fester (from *The Adams Family* to describe women's bald head), Easter Chick (to describe the soft, fuzzy nature of their hair as it grew in), and Groucho Marx (to describe a daughter's eyebrows, as one brow grew back growing upward and the other brow was growing downward). Some women even had nicknames for their tumors and breasts (e.g., Frankenboob) that were removed.

Other women recalled finding humor in unexpected situations. They noted that humor functioned adaptively by lightening up the serious nature of the cancer experience. For example, one mother-daughter dyad recalled joking every time the daughter's 3-year-old son put on her wig. Another mother-daughter pair focused on the "ridiculousness" of the cancer experience. This daughter recalled that she frequently experienced side effects that were considered less common (e.g., losing eyelashes after chemotherapy). She and her mother reportedly used humor to cope with these extreme bodily changes:

> I was one of those freaks that "Oh, this hardly ever happens to anyone that all their eyelashes fall off." You know what I mean? I was always like the exception so it became a joke. We kicked about it. You know, like I always say, "You know what? It's still not as bad as having both your breasts removed!" That just became the joke. (21b)

In addition, a daughter recalled that she and her mother joked about their experiences with menopause. This daughter experienced chemotherapy-induced menopause, and her mother happened to be going through natural menopause at the exact same time. This mother and daughter were even taking the same medication. The diagnosed daughter went into detail about how she and her mother laughed together about their side effects, especially the hot flashes. Exhibiting the humor, she said, "We *love* being in menopause together!" (14b).

Lifting Me Up

Mothers often made special efforts to cheer up their daughters throughout their cancer experience. These efforts included sending funny cards, care packages, flowers, and books. Daughters also recalled that they especially appreciated it when their mothers took them out to lunch or dinner. Several daughters recalled that this type of support helped them feel better able to deal with the disease.

This type of emotional support communication tied particularly to daughters' treatment experiences. Mothers often sent their daughters things to cheer them up when they had a lot of "down time" at home alone as a result of being in treatment. For instance, some mothers sent their daughters care packages or funny notes. They also often accompanied their daughters to treatment sessions. One daughter recalled, "Right after my first chemo treatment, we went out to lunch and we got a manicure/pedicure. [She laughs.] Then she took me shopping!" (22b).

Mothers further enacted this emotional support by doing things to celebrate various milestones throughout the cancer experience (e.g., the end of treatment). Both mothers and daughters felt that celebrations lifted their emotional state. Some daughters even celebrated with formal trips abroad or to the beach with their entire families to commemorate key points in their cancer experience. One mother recalled several celebrations that were instrumental in cheering her daughter up:

> Her friends had a benefit for her right before she entered treatment. . . . That was enormously uplifting for her. . . . And then after she finished treatment it was her birthday, and we arranged a hall and we had a birthday party for her. And she really enjoyed that! (33a).

ENACTED SUPPORT THAT FUNCTIONS BOTH ADAPTIVELY AND MALADAPTIVELY

Some supportive communication that daughters experienced with their mothers functioned adaptively at times but maladaptively at others. Whether support helped daughters cope seemed inherently tied to developmental issues for the daughter—challenges that are particularly salient in the mother-daughter bond at this point in the daughter's adulthood.

Being There

Daughters and their mothers frequently stated that the most helpful enacted support daughters received from their mothers was simply "being there." Mothers often expressed this support verbally by telling their daughters that they were there for them no matter what. As one mother stated, "Many times I've said, 'You've got me, and I've got you'" (13a). When mothers could not physically be there for their daughters (e.g., during surgeries), they often verbally expressed that they were "there" with them in spirit. Some women even told their daughters to do things to remind them that they were there with them. For example, one told her daughter to squeeze her own hand to symbolize the mother's presence.

Daughters also described consistently having a sense or feeling that their mothers were "there" for them. For them, the expression meant they could rely on their mothers in coping with breast cancer. The sense that their mothers were there for them seemed to put daughters at peace. As one stated, "I would say it made it easier—the fact that she was by my side. . . . My mother was by my side" (22b). Another daughter stated, "She always did what she said she was going to do. I could always count on her" (21b). Interestingly, when asked, many mothers admitted that they rarely asked their daughters if it was okay to "be there." Rather, they merely assumed that their daughters wanted them to enact this type of support or that it was the right thing to do.

"Being there" typically referred to supportive communication in two contexts: health advocacy/partnership or companionship. First, diagnosed women discussed this form of communication in relation to their mothers being present in the health setting. Some mothers acted as their daughters' advocates in doctors' appointments and during treatment. One daughter described how her mother enacted the support of "being there" in this context:

> She took a very big part of being my partner. She made sure she was there with my first—when I first sat down with the doctor to talk about the type of cancer I had. . . . And she would always drive me to my chemo treatments. She set the standard for everyone else. (13b)

The participants reported numerous types of behavior their mothers enacted in the health setting that conveyed to them that their mothers were emotionally supporting them by "being there." For instance, some mothers helped their daughters remember questions to ask doctors and also listened and talked to them about medical decisions. Mothers seemed to feel that being there in this context was important, particularly if the daughter was not married. As one mother stated, "[Me being there] is having someone to share it with, because she's by herself" (38a).

The adaptive functioning of mothers "being there" as a health advocate or partner depended on certain factors. "Being there" functioned adaptively when daughters and mothers worked together in the health setting. As one mother indicated:

> We go to the doctor's. I go with her and she talks and then I ask questions. And a lot of times she'll have me write things down for her so she can have a record of it. . . . They gave a whole lot of information and, you know, there are so many questions. We just wrote them all down and we looked at the question. And so I had the questions and I would ask [her] "Is it okay?" to make sure because I think when anyone goes to the doctor in a situation like that, they could be telling you stuff but you don't really hear it or you can't remember. (22a)

Daughters seemed to appreciate their mother's advocacy in this sense. Many noted that support in this context was helpful because the experience was so shocking. They recalled that because of the shock, it can be difficult to remember everything health professionals say during appointments. This adaptive functioning of "being there" in health interactions was especially helpful during chemotherapy treatment when daughters struggled with "chemo fog" or "chemo brain," a side effect that adversely affects short-term memory. One daughter pointed out:

> Chemotherapy kind of gives you a bit of a brain fog, they call it, and sometimes you forget things and can't remember things that are told to you. So you really need somebody there that will listen to what the doctor or whomever is saying and if you forget, to be able to tell you . . . and getting them to explain the treatment and when I have had problems with the treatment to, you know, try helping me speak to the doctor or person in charge to get things changed for the better. (13b)

"Being there" in the health setting also functioned maladaptively at times. This occurred when mothers asked too many questions, became emotional or confused, or neglected to negotiate their role with the daughter. In these circumstances, the mother's presence became a source of distress for daughters. When this was the case, most daughters did not invite their mothers to future medical appointments or treatments. One daughter shared such an experience:

> She went along to the initial appointment where they told me what stage it was and things like that and it really, really upset her and she was really confused. So then I didn't want her to go to the appointments like that because I just thought it was too upsetting for her. . . . I had mixed emotions [about her coming]. . . . I think it was more stressful. . . . She hung on certain words they said. . . . Sometimes she makes me a little more nervous when she's in there 'cause she'll ask too many questions. . . . She'll drive me crazy like just picking or something, you know like nagging me. Like "Oh did you do this? Or you need to ask them what? Why is this?" (34b)

Mothers often recognized when "being there" was not emotionally supportive or helpful to their daughters' adjustment to cancer. For instance, they seemed aware that, at times, they asked too many questions. However, even though they were concerned about the consequences of this behavior, not all mothers associated it with why their daughters eventually shut them out or monitored their involvement in the health setting. It also seemed particularly important for mothers to negotiate their role with their daughters for "being there" to function adaptively in the health setting. For instance, a daughter recalled finding out that her mother was asking her physician questions without her knowing. She mentioned being upset with her mother's behavior and feeling frustrated about her mother's inability to understand why she was upset. She expressed her frustration, saying, "I understand that I am her daughter, but you still shouldn't be having conversations with my doctor about me. . . . And again, I was wrong for thinking there was anything wrong with that!" (33b).

The second context in which women characterized their mothers as "being there" was when their mothers provided them companionship—usually in daughters' homes. The adaptive functioning of this type of support depended on a number of factors. Daughters indicated that having their mothers there made them feel less alone. They also felt that having their mothers with them in their homes gave them something other than their condition on which to focus. As one daughter stated, "It was nice to have [her] around too and nice to have the company when you're just kind of laying on the couch all day" (15b). Daughters' mothers seemed to want to be there as well. One mother said, "[I was] wanting to make sure I was with her all the time, didn't want her by herself, you know? Just listening to her talk, her concerns . . ." (38a). Often the mothers were thrilled that their daughters wanted to spend time together, particularly when they perceived their daughters as characteristically independent.

When this enacted support functioned adaptively, these instances were times in which daughters *wanted* their mothers' companionship. One, whose mother came and stayed with her, noted wanting her mother there while she underwent treatment. She recalled how therapeutic their companionship was for her:

> When I was done with treatment it was kind of depressing because we didn't have these sleepovers anymore. . . . We'd stay up those nights when she slept over. We'd stay up those nights and talk. But not necessarily about the whole cancer thing. I think it was more like camaraderie. You know, like old times type of thing [reminiscing]. . . . It made us feel more—well, you always feel good when you talk to your family about the way things were, like there's a part of your childhood that helps make up who you are and I think when you bring those feelings back, then I guess it's like healing in a way. (21b)

"Being there" as a daughter's companion also seemed to function more adaptively when the women respected each other's space. As one daughter stated, "Sometimes you just want to be alone." On occasion both mothers and daughters seemed to be aware of one another's need for space. One mother recalled that it was often difficult to leave her daughter, but that it was necessary. She reflected on a time in which she left her daughter alone for an extended period to visit another ailing family member:

> I didn't want to go anywhere without her . . . because for all these past months, she's been right there beside me. And I feel like if she's with

> me, then everything is okay because I know she's okay. . . . It did me good [to leave her daughter alone] and it did her good. Gave her some, you know, a little bit of alone time and it gave me some. (13a)

Mothers noted that they eventually gave their daughters more and more space when they seemed to be feeling better, were ending treatment, or were not bothered by being alone.

Space was important in whether "being there" as a companion functioned adaptively. When mothers did not give their daughters space, their companionship was not helpful in their adjustment to the disease. At times mothers' presence competed with their daughters' husbands' presence. Other times too much time together resulted in personality clashes, as one mother observed:

> The trouble is I think, we're a lot alike, and you know how that is. You can just go at each other. And then I'll tell her, "I think it's time for me to go home and are you feeling okay and good enough? If not, I'll stay." (34a)

Daughters also described a need for space but for different reasons. They described feeling responsible for their mothers being there. Also, some daughters felt they could sense their mothers' emotions about the disease. Even if they wanted their mothers with them, sometimes the mothers stayed too long. As one daughter stated when her mother was leaving after an extended stay, "I'm ready to have my space back!" (15b).

Consistency also contributed to whether support functioned adaptively in either the health setting or as a daughter's companion. When mothers were not consistently "there" for their daughters, they questioned their mothers' priorities. Some even felt that their mothers were not putting their feelings and needs first. Several daughters discussed situations they believed conveyed to them that their mothers were only "half" there. Interestingly, all of these experiences occurred during the daughters' treatment of surgery or chemotherapy. These daughters all made reference to moments when their mothers gave greater priority to their own feelings and needs or their siblings' rather than their daughters'. In these daughters' experiences, the mother had been conveying to the daughter that she was "there" (e.g., being there at the daughter's appointments, in her home, or at the hospital). However, the mother then abruptly pulled away. Some daughters, for instance, talked about their mothers going on unplanned vacations during their treatment. One did so right after the daughter's first chemotherapy treatment. Daughters also recalled their mothers putting their siblings' needs ahead of their own. In these cases, daughters felt their mothers disregarded their feelings or the seriousness of their experience by prioritizing the needs of a sibling. One daughter described feeling like, "I can't even have cancer!" (21b). When daughters interpreted their mother's supportive behavior as inconsistent, they also perceived the behavior as odd and confusing.

Mothers rarely mentioned such experiences. When they did, it was in reference to the daughters' experiences with their siblings. These mothers also mentioned that they still struggled with trying not to give greater priority to one child's needs, even when one daughter had cancer. As one mother explained, "I have two. I try to keep it equal. It's hard to do that sometimes" (33a).

Mothering

Mothers also enacted emotional support by "mothering" their daughters. Many of the daughters felt that the diagnosis increased their mothers' maternal behavior. Daughters made sense of this change in behavior as their mothers' maternal instinct kicking in. One woman described this support in saying:

> It seems like they go into doting mode. They want to be the first ones there. They want to be there to know everything, to help. And I think they just go into that mode where they need to fix it and they can't. (34b)

Mothering consisted of calling daughters to check in on them (often every day), asking them questions to make sure they were taking care of themselves, and trying to be helpful. One daughter characterized her mother's "doting" as follows:

> Oh my God! She would make sure I was eating or try to eat or drink. "Have you drank today? Did you drink water? You have to drink something. You know you have to drink something. Did you take your meds?" It was a typical mom situation kind of thing like when your kid is sick. (14b)

Women differed by relationship in terms of how much mothering they experienced. However, the daughters typically perceived that the mothering support was tied to the mother wanting to be of assistance (e.g., come over to help in any way), providing comfort (e.g., being affectionate), and making sure they were doing okay (e.g., calling frequently to check in on them).

Whether this behavior functioned adaptively or maladaptively in emotionally supporting daughters depended on the daughters' perceptions of whether the support was excessive. The daughters noted that their mothers' calls and questions let them know they were concerned about them. Many diagnosed women shared this expressed concern was comforting. However, others felt that when the calls and questions were too frequent, mothering communication was not helpful. Several daughters admitted this type of support could even become annoying. One daughter described feeling that it was important that mothers not "overdo it" or overreact:

> She was calling, calling, calling constantly. I totally understand that she was worried or whatever. It did get annoying after a while and I'm like "Mom I'm fine. . . . I will call if I'm not fine." . . . It was like every day and drove me insane every single day. And I'm like, "Oh my God! I'm fine!" . . . I said, "Mom, you don't have to call every day." [She said] "I don't care. I just want to make sure you're okay." I'm like, "Mom I'm fine. If I'm not going to be fine, I will call you." (14b)

When daughters felt the mothering support was excessive, they mentioned becoming upset with their mothers and even cutting conversations short. Some mothers seemed to understand daughters' need to not be overmothered. One mother who lived some distance from her daughter described being careful not to overdo the mothering support of calling to check in:

> I'd just check in periodically. . . . I have to remember, too, that she's not feeling well this day [treatment days]. I mean, I think I would phone when I knew she was having a treatment or whatever. I'd phone a couple of days later to give her a chance to recoup a little bit and then see how things were. Or, you know, I'd phone [her daughter's husband] when she was in the hospital and stuff and see how things were and stuff like that. But I wasn't on the phone [a lot]. I kept thinking, you know, when you're sick, the last thing you want is 50 million people phoning you to see how you're doing, even if it is your mother. (15a)

Daughters' experiences also suggested that a sense of control was a key factor in whether they found the mothering to be helpful. For mothering to function adaptively, daughters seemed to want some control of their mothers' support. For example, it was important for daughters to determine whether and when they needed their mothers' help. This sense of control seemed especially important because daughters felt such a loss of control because of their medical condition. Daughters noted feeling torn between understanding their mothers' need to mother them and a need for control themselves because the disease had robbed them of so much control over their lives. One daughter summed up this dilemma:

> I think it was just—it was hard for her just because here her daughter has cancer. She wants to be there and help her. And me, I like to be independent and I don't like to ask for help from people. So that made it hard for her because you know she is living at a distance. I think—she sat there [and thought], "I want to be there for my daughter. And I want to help her and here she is fighting me on it." You know what I mean? But you know when you're diagnosed with cancer you lose that sense of control over your own body yourself, and any little bit of control or independence you can have you want. So that makes it hard. (34b)

The daughters' dialectical struggles with feelings of control, with respect to whether mothering functioned adaptively or maladaptively, depended on whether the mothers respected their daughters' need to call the shots. For instance, one daughter recalled her mother being fine with her not answering the phone when her mother called to check in on her. On these occasions, she simply left the message that she wanted to see how the daughter was and to give her a call when she could. Another daughter recalled her mother allowing her to decide whether she needed her:

> I like it in that she will offer, "Whatever you need. Just tell me." But not you know—not pushy about it. Not "Oh I want to come down there. I'm coming down. I'm taking care of you!" You know she never did that. So she sort of left it up to me, and I liked that. I was sort of like, "Okay, I actually need you to come down now." [And she responded] "Okay, yeah. I'll do it and I'll figure out what to tell them [at work] that I'm not working that week." . . . So yeah I had asked her and she was really happy when I asked. She wanted to be wanted that way and didn't want to impose that on me and ask. . . . So she was really excited. (15b)

Staying Positive

Women described various forms of enacted emotional support from their mothers that centered on their remaining positive in their outlook as they struggled with body image, lost their hair, expressed distressing emotions, or waited for test results. Although mothers admitted that talking positively to their daughters was sometimes difficult, as they too felt the strain of coping with cancer, they felt it was nonetheless necessary. Many of the daughters also shared that mothers' positivity was critical to their adjustment and survival.

Mothers engaged in positive talk in many ways, including reassurance, encouragement, being optimistic, and maintaining a positive attitude when they talked with their daughters. They also told their daughters stories of other survivors to reassure them. They sometimes complemented their daughters for how strong they were, how beautiful they looked during treatment and hair loss, and how proud they were of them. Mothers recalled that positive talk was important in "pumping up" daughters when they seemed down. As one mother stated, "If you had a positive attitude, you could come through a lot of things. And without one, sometimes they just didn't make it" (13a). Several mothers noted the importance of this quality on multiple levels. One mother recalled the power of her daughter's positivity on her own attitude:

> I remember her saying once when she went to the cancer clinic and they had a group and they put her in. And she said, "I was probably one of the youngest ones there." She says, "But there was this one lady there." And she says, "I just felt so bad for her, Mom, because I just really felt like she wasn't going to make it because of her attitude. Like she was so whiney, and it was almost like she wasn't fighting. You know, you've got to fight! You can't say, 'Why me?' You've got to say, 'Hey, it's me!'" [My daughter's] positive attitude has made my attitude better. (15a)

Some daughters felt that being positive was how they and their families approached life. One daughter bluntly stated that it was an outlook of "Shit happens. . . . Get over it" (14b). Many women also felt that any negative talk was pointless, saying, "You're in it for the long haul. There's no turning back" (15a). Daughters seemed to feel their mothers shared this outlook, and that positive talk was behavior they jointly enacted. According to one daughter:

> It's both of us. . . . I think we always try to take something good out of it. Let's just look at it, see where it's taking us, where can we go with it, and hopefully we come out a better person after it. (21b)

In contrast, some daughters recalled that their mothers' positive behavior ran counter to the norm. Regardless of whether the positive talk was new for mothers and daughters, for the most part, positive talk was often helpful in daughters' adjustment. The mothers' enacted support helped minimize their anxiety and gave them hope. Mothers also often recognized that their positive talk helped minimize their daughters' worries. One daughter recalled how she worried about test results she was waiting on. She felt that when her mother responded positively, it was helpful:

> I say, "You know I talked to [the hospital]. They said this." She may say "Oh that's great! That's good news!" Or I'll get her opinion on something, like "Oh so what do you think? Do you think everything's going to be okay?" And she's like, "Oh yeah. I don't have any bad feelings. I think things are going to be fine." She is positive in that sense and sometimes I'm like "Are you just saying that?" You know? It's so unusual for her! [She laughs]. . . . She'll tell me not to worry about something, which is surprising coming from her. But if I say, "Oh my gosh! I got to go through this test. I hope everything's okay. Oh my gosh! I hope it doesn't come back!" And she'll be like, "[Daughter's name], don't even worry! Everything's going to be fine. You'll be fine. If it is something, we'll deal with it." . . . Sometimes I just need to hear that. (34b)

Some women admitted that, although they appreciated the positive talk from their mothers, at times they took their mothers' words with a "grain of salt." In these instances, daughters admitted that nothing could make them feel better. This experience often coincided with daughters' loss of hair or struggle with body image after a surgery. For example, after her mastectomy, one daughter reflected on feeling "free" to choose clothes more easily because she was no longer large breasted. However, at the same time, she had difficulties adjusting to her new body:

> I remember going out to some mall. . . . I had always been kind of top heavy. It was weird for me to be flat. . . . I was like [to my mother], "Everybody has boobs!" and I just kind of like put it out there. And she was like, "You will be getting well again soon." . . . I don't know if there's anything she can say that was really helpful. . . . I was feeling bad. . . . I had to just kind of work it out on my own so I don't think that she handled it like good or bad or anything—I don't know if there's anything she could really do. (38b)

Positive talk functioned maladaptively when daughters felt that their mothers were also being dismissive of their feelings. As one stated, "As long as it's just talking positive and not crossing over [my feelings], it's helpful. Once [she] crosses over something, then it's not helpful." In this case, the daughter recalled her mother minimizing her concerns about recurrence. "Sometimes she goes, 'You don't really have to worry about that because you're young, and your doctors are on top of things'" (13b). Another daughter described a similar experience when she expressed her frustration over trying to find a bathing suit that fit her after her mastectomy:

> I have a big divot under my arm [from the surgery]. And the first time I went bathing suit shopping, I was with my mom, and that was one time I remember [her saying], "Well it doesn't look too bad." And I'm standing there. I came home bawling. I was really—that really upset me. Because that's when it really hit me that this was—bathing suits are not made for people without breasts. . . . I think that was one of those [instances] where you don't understand. Like I remember saying to her she didn't understand because she wasn't the one going through it. . . . I needed to talk to someone else who went through it. (21b)

These daughters felt their mothers' positive talk minimized their emotions or concerns. As a result, their mothers' communicative support was unhelpful in their adjustment. One mother's reflection indicated that it may be necessary for mothers to respond in a way that allows daughters to express both positive and negative emotions. She talked about this when describing her own daughter's struggles with adjusting to cancer:

> Sometimes when she was down [and I was] trying to convince her that it was going to be okay, you know, it was going to get better. I think sometimes she was very, very tired and down. . . . You know, you can't go through something like that and not have the ups and downs. (13a)

Validating Decisions

Daughters also needed their mothers' validation. This type of enacted emotional support communication was most important when daughters shared their treatment decisions with their mothers. As previously noted in Chapter 9, daughters often told their mothers about their care decisions (e.g., whether to have a mastectomy) *after* they had made them. Hence, daughters were not looking for their mothers' input. They were not sharing their decisions in an effort to talk through them. Daughters noted that in these instances, if their mothers validated their decisions, this support was especially helpful in their adjustment to breast cancer.

Mothers enacted validation by reaffirming daughters' decisions, agreeing with them, not questioning their decisions, and not suggesting what they should do. It was especially important for daughters to feel that their mothers had faith in their decisions. One daughter said, "She just always, you know, believes exactly what I believe and is totally behind how I feel about everything and you know, just knows that I am strong" (15b). Mothers admitted not always agreeing with their daughters' decisions. However, they rarely voiced this. Instead, they told their daughters that they believed in what they were doing. One mother reflected on her reasons for doing so even when she felt her daughter should make a different decision:

> She had all the facts, and she knew what all the consequences were. And she had the facts and like nobody—I don't think anyone can know what they would do if they were in that exact position unless they were in that position 'cause she had the facts and all the information. . . . It's her choice. (22a)

Sometimes daughters received validation from their mothers after they followed through with decisions (e.g., having a mastectomy or getting genetic testing). Other women's mothers expressed their validation beforehand. When mothers enacted this support, daughters felt it helped in adjusting to living with cancer because this response did not burden them with underlying pressure; it minimized their negative emotions, and it showed them that their mothers believed in them. As one daughter stated:

> She just kept it real simple and said, "Yeah, you know, whatever you think you need to do" or "That makes sense—whatever makes sense to you." . . . She was never like, "Well, you know, you really should do" [or] "I understand how you feel, but you know this is why you should do that." . . . You never felt like there was this underlying pressure from somebody. (15b)

Another daughter recalled that it was important that her mother never questioned her decisions because questioning would have added to her negative distress. This woman recalled how hard it was to adjust to her hair loss, and in an effort to adapt, she invested in several wigs. She recalled how her mother's validation helped her adjust:

> [She] never questions why would I be spending money on wigs, which I am glad because I am kind of [feeling] guilty, like I shouldn't be spending money. It was like one of the things I just needed to do. (38b)

For this supportive behavior to even be enacted by mothers, it was critical that they understood that their daughters were not asking them for their insight when they openly talked about their medical decisions. Several mothers seemed to comprehend this as one mother summed up:

> She was just talking to me, saying, "These are my options, and I don't like this option, and I would prefer not to do this if I didn't have to.

> And I'm going to look into it some more and see what else I can do." You know, things like that. I don't think she was asking my permission. . . . I've always said, "You know what? It's your body. You know your body better than anybody. And it's your mind too." . . . If you are not comfortable with it, it's not going to be good for you. . . . It wasn't a matter of saying, "Oh what do you think of this?" It was a matter of, "This is what I'm looking at right now." (15a)

When mothers did not understand this need, they did not demonstrate faith in their daughters' decisions. Consequently, their responses negatively affected the daughters' adjustment. Ultimately, a lack of validation (and even disagreeing with daughters' decisions) resulted in daughters withdrawing from their mothers. Daughters recalled that when their mothers did not validate their decisions, they cut them off in conversation, changed the subject, or refrained from talking to their mothers about their decisions in the future. Behavior that functioned maladaptively in this context included the mothers questioning their daughters' decisions (e.g., "Are you sure?"), arguing with them about decisions, or letting the daughters know they opposed the decision. For instance, one daughter recalled her mother not agreeing with her when she decided to have a mastectomy instead of a lumpectomy. The daughter felt her decision was appropriate because it gave her the "best shot" at survival. This woman recalled her mother arguing with her on other decisions as well. She eventually completely shut her mother out of any of her breast cancer experience. Interestingly, mothers in these cases seemed to be aware that their daughters were not seeking their permission and that their opinions did not motivate their daughters' decisions. Nonetheless, they sometimes continued to engage in what the daughter perceived as non-validating communication.

13

DAUGHTERS AND MOTHERS COPING IN MIDLIFE

I wanted to know what she was doing . . . that made me feel comfortable to know if she was continuing to go, you know, out to lunch with friends or going to her study groups and all that. I wanted to know that she continued on and wasn't sitting there dwelling on me or anything else. . . . For her to continue her life as she is, that's actually, that's comforting to me. That makes me feel the comfort I need to do what I need to do. . . . That actually brings me so much comfort. I can sit here and do what I need to do for myself and not be worried about her. I can concentrate on myself more so.
Diagnosed Midlife Mother

Just kind of a realization that she's not going to be here forever on my part made me want to call her and talk to her more. . . . I think my mom needed me to be there for her. . . . And I needed to talk to her because I was scared and didn't know what was going to happen. . . . I'll just call her when I'm walking home from class just to say hi and tell her about my day and see how she's doing and stuff like that. And I would never do that before. I would never even think about it. . . . I think it's a combination of the [breast cancer] and me growing up a little bit. Mostly I

think the change is in me than in her. Because I think she always wanted this kind of relationship with me, and I've just never kind of been willing to give it until now.
Daughter of a Diagnosed Midlife Mother

I think just knowing that she's there . . . no matter what, she'll do it if she can. . . . It's not something you can put your arms around or define, and it's always been there. She always told me, "If there is anything that you can give to your child, it's something I hope I've given to you, is I'm always there."
Diagnosed Midlife Daughter

I've learned from experience. I am 70 years old. I've learned from experience that it doesn't do any good to think about it and sit around and mope. You have to get up and go out and do something to make you feel better.
Mother of a Diagnosed Midlife Daughter

DIAGNOSED MIDLIFE DAUGHTERS AND THEIR MOTHERS

The "juggling act" of midlife did not stop for these diagnosed women who often described non-emotional forms of support as critical to their well-being and disease adjustment. While these daughters and mothers did not necessarily openly share emotional aspects of disease coping, they exhibited an intuitive sense of how to be there for one another.

ADAPTIVE ENACTED EMOTIONAL SUPPORT

Like the previous age group of diagnosed daughters, two of types of emotional support (*listening* and *being humorous*) also surfaced as behaviors that were always helpful to midlife diagnosed women's disease adjustment. However, middle-adult daughter-mother dyads described the support type of *being there* differently and as always helpful (thus, adaptive) in their shared coping. The adaptive nature of these forms of support are embedded within the cancer-related context of various stressors that diagnosed women faced.

Being There

Midlife daughters frequently shared that their mother was most emotionally supportive to them by just "being there." This included mothers being physically present during surgery and treatment. However, unlike young-adult-diagnosed daughter-mother dyads, their presence entailed only physical presence, not serving as a health advocate or partner in fighting cancer. None of the mothers appeared to be involved in doctor-patient discussions (with the exception of one mother who was also a nurse), and most were there just to "be" with their daughters or keep them company. Women recalled knowing that their mothers did not want them to be alone, whether it was at an appointment, treatment, or even at home.

The diagnosed women also described "being there" in relation to being present in the daughters' home during treatment and recovery. Some mothers even moved in with their daughters for an extended time period. At times the mothers seemed to be most helpful in instrumental forms of support (e.g., housework, helping with the daughters' children, and caregiving for daughters while healing). This finding is noteworthy. Even though diagnosed daughters were consistently asked about helpful emotionally focused support, they tended to focus most on instrumental forms of support (as it is defined in scholarship). Some stated that this form of support was most helpful and important to them or what they needed most to adjust. Instrumental support may have overshadowed emotional forms given midlife is a time when women are "juggling" the most responsibilities, oftentimes as a mother, daughter to aging parents, professional, wife or spouse, and friend. Managing day-to-day life was likely a more pressing issue that diagnosed midlife women needed assistance with.

Like young-adult daughters, women in midlife also frequently referred to "being there" as a nonverbal, unspoken sense of presence that allowed them to know their mothers would be available in any way and at any time they needed. Daughters described this form of support as something they knew they could constantly rely on. For instance, one daughter noted how her mother created this intuitive sense of "being there" to support her as she adjusted to breast cancer:

> I think just knowing that she's there. . . . Knowing that I can count on her. And no matter what, she'll do it if she can. . . . It's not something you can put your arms around or define, and it's always been there. It's not something new. . . . It was always there. . . . She always told me, "If there is anything you can give to your child, it's something I hope I've given to you, is I'm always there." (11b)

Daughters seemed to feel that having their mothers "there" brought them comfort and made them feel loved. Most daughters observed that this communication was how their mothers always supported them. These daughters said something like, "That's just her." Only one daughter felt the behavior was out of the norm. Nonetheless, she too welcomed her mother's "being there" support and said that it helped her adjust. She recalled this experience, saying, "She really wanted to be here. . . . She wanted to be around. . . . I don't usually see a tender side of her, and that was probably the closest thing to it. And that was kind of special" (35b). Many women also indicated that they felt this form of support was helpful for mothers' adjustment as well as theirs. These daughters believed that allowing their mothers to "be there" for them helped the mother feel more at ease with her daughter's condition and well-being. Daughters may have understood this maternal need or were more in tune to it given most were mothers themselves.

Often daughters reported that they never had to ask their mothers for anything or tell them to "be there." Rather, the mothers just undertook this support at their initiative. Additionally, mothers often admitted that their daughters never asked them to be there for them. Daughters sometimes told their mothers that it was not necessary for them to be there physically. Some mothers did as their daughters told them, but other mothers joined them anyway. Daughters seemed to accept and appreciate this. As one daughter explained, "She just wanted to be there."

Being Willing to Listen

Like younger diagnosed daughters, midlife daughters felt that their mothers' listening support was helpful in their ability to adjust to the diagnosis. Women in this cohort described their mothers' listening behavior as "being a sounding board" when they needed to talk. Hence, this form of communicated emotional support seemed partially connected to daughters' intuitive sense that their mothers were there for them (i.e., *being there*).

As in the young-adult dyads, diagnosed daughters in the middle adulthood group referred to their mothers enacting this type of support when they voiced their fears of getting through it, which was not something they typically disclosed or did more than once. Some also felt that listening was important when they shared with their mothers the medical decisions they had made. By mothers listening to them, the daughters felt that their mothers "accepted" their decisions. Many described this support as helpful *any* time they needed to talk. One daughter said, "She didn't always have all the right words or sometimes she didn't even answer me. She just listened to what I had to say, and that was okay" (11b).

Being Humorous

Interviewees also recalled that humor was adaptive in their adjustment. They noted that this form of support consisted of talking about funny memories they had experienced over the course of the cancer, saying goofy things, as well as talking about funny television shows. One mother recalled periodically sending her daughter cute cartoons to lift her spirits. Although this type of support was not as prominently experienced in these women's lives as in the younger group of dyads, it nevertheless seemed to lighten the air of the cancer experience in the same adaptive manner. One mother felt that this was important in her daughter's mental well-being, saying, "I was just trying to keep her spirits up . . . [and] brighten her day" (10a).

ENACTED SUPPORT THAT FUNCTIONS BOTH ADAPTIVELY AND MALADAPTIVELY

Like the younger cohort of bonds, *mothering* and *staying positive* functioned both adaptively and maladaptively. Middle-adulthood daughters' descriptions varied slightly from the younger dyads' experiences, however, exhibiting more of an intuitive sense of each other's needs and motives in enacting these forms of support.

Mothering

Daughters acknowledged "mothering" as a form of emotional support that included calling to check in daily (or quite frequently) in addition to asking the daughter questions in a mothering way (e.g., Are you eating? Are you getting enough rest?). The daughters saw this type of support as indicative of an increased focus on their health and a heightened concern mothers had in making sure their daughters were doing okay. They sometimes described this support as their mother's "way." They also seemed to understand that when mothers supported them in this manner, the mothers believed they were doing something to help their daughters. In turn, mothers were cognizant of the fact that they were emotionally supporting their daughter by enacting "mothering" communication. They admitted that they were especially worried about their daughters. One mother, noting that it could function maladaptively, stated, "I might have hovered a little bit more than maybe she wanted me to, but she never voiced it. Sometimes you have to back off a little too" (11b).

Most believed that this behavior helped daughters adjust. For instance, one daughter talked about how "mothering" encouraged her to take care of herself. She admitted that when her mother asked her whether she was getting enough rest, exercising, and eating right, she tended to watch what she ate or tried to manage stress better. Other daughters seemed simply to accept this type of support and, at the same time, appreciate it. Their acceptance could be linked to the fact that the daughters understood its importance to their mothers' adjustment. As evident in their description of "being there," daughters felt this type of support was also helpful to their mothers' well-being. They needed to "mother" their daughters. More than half the daughters had children of their own (compared with only two of the diagnosed young-adult daughters), which may account, in part, for their increased understanding of their mothers' need to "mother" them.

Only a couple of daughters mentioned how the behavior functioned maladaptively. Ultimately, like young-adult-diagnosed daughters' experiences, mothering was not helpful when their mothers overdid it. One woman indicated how the behavior sometimes made her feel abnormal and like something was wrong with her. Mothering seemed to convey to her that she was to be pitied. Another daughter reported being irritated. She shared her experience with her 80-year-old mother's behavior and how she overdid it:

> She always calls me and checks up on me. . . . And if she doesn't get me, I mean she'll freak and she'll start calling my friends. And so literally I have to tell her where I am at all times. . . . It was a little excessive. . . . I don't care that she checks in on me, but she can't panic if she can't find me. (5b)

Although such maladaptive functioning was consistent with young-adult dyads' experiences, midlife daughters typically framed this support as helpful. Moreover, they frequently revealed an understanding of the mothers' need to engage in this behavior in order to enhance their own sense of wellness.

Staying Positive

Daughters often discussed positive talk as a way their mothers emotionally supported them like other cohorts. This type of support included their mothers verbally encouraging them, reassuring them, and complimenting them on how they were doing. Mothers encouraged their daughters to keep fighting or reassured them they were coping well. They also reassured their daughters when they disclosed fears or concerns about what could happen in the future. Daughters felt that their mothers talked positively throughout the cancer experience. Sometimes mothers provided this type of support when daughters were feeling "yucky" from treatment side effects.

Daughters noted that this type of talk was helpful in their adjustment. As one explained, "She was very, very positive and very upbeat right away. . . . That was a really good thing to hear right off the bat" (10b). Mothers also admitted trying to point out "the positives" and always maintain a positive atmosphere. One mother mentioned her firm belief in enacting this type of emotional support:

> I've learned from experience. I am 70 years old, and I've learned from experience that it doesn't do any good to think about it and sit around and mope. You know, you have to get up and go out and do something to make you feel better. (7a)

These descriptions seemed to mirror young-adult daughter-mother dyads' experiences. However, women in the middle adulthood dyads did talk about one form of communicative behavior that conveyed positivity those in the younger age group did not—reframing. Mothers often reframed situations their daughters encountered in a more positive light. According to the daughters, they felt their mothers' ability to reframe situations was particularly helpful in their adjustment. For instance, one mother reframed her daughter's anxiety about the diagnosis (the "what ifs") by telling her to focus only on what they knew for sure. Another mother reframed her daughter's complaints about her husband (who was not helping with the children and housework during her chemotherapy treatment) by telling her of situations that could be worse. A third mother reframed the seriousness of her daughter's disease by focusing on how happy she was that the diagnosis was not terminal (a revelation she had after the Virginia Tech tragedy occurred). All of these instances of reframing seemed to help daughters rethink how they were doing and made them feel better about their situations.

Although the daughters frequently talked about how helpful positivity was in their adjustment, two situations indicated that talking positively may not be helpful at times. One daughter mentioned not really wanting to hear her mother's positive talk when she was feeling bad from treatment side effects. She just wanted to "lay there." Another daughter said that initially her mother's positivity made her feel as if she did not realize how serious the situation was. She reported this response: "I think my initial reaction to her being so positive was almost like, 'No it's not! What do you mean? How can you think like that?'" (10b). These situations are similar to the younger dyads' recollections of how positive talk is not always adaptive. For midlife-diagnosed daughters, positive talk was not helpful when it simultaneously minimized or dismissed daughters' present or "in-the-moment" feelings and concerns.

DIAGNOSED MIDLIFE MOTHERS AND THEIR DAUGHTERS

When midlife-diagnosed women described their emotional support experiences with their daughters, their illustrations were extremely positive in nature compared with other age groups. Hence, their stories are more heavily focused on adaptive rather than maladaptive communication. Moreover, these diagnosed women were often more concerned with how their daughters were responding to their illness. As such, what these mothers perceived as helpful support in their own disease coping was very much tied to whether it helped the daughter cope as well.

ADAPTIVE ENACTED EMOTIONAL SUPPORT

Five types of support characterized previous dyads' experiences. However, a new form (*staying normal*) important to women's adjustment emerged for midlife-diagnosed mothers. In sync with the previous two age groups of dyads, *listening*, *showing affection*, and *being humorous* always functioned adaptively. Unlike young-adult-diagnosed daughters, but consistent with midlife-diagnosed daughters' reports, *being there* always functioned in a helpful manner. Interestingly, unlike the other dyads, the current cohort of women felt that *staying positive* was always helpful emotional support.

Being Willing to Listen

As in other mother-daughter dyads, it was important to mothers in this group that their daughters listen to them. They were not very descriptive in characterizing this form of emotional support, however. Typically, they simply reported that it was important to them that "she just listened" (30a) or that "listening was helpful" (39a). At times the support elicited an empathetic response (e.g., "I'm sorry you feel this way") or a positive comment (e.g., "Things will get better"). More commonly, mothers and daughters described this behavior without reference to any verbalizations on the daughters' part.

Daughters often talked about providing this type of support because they did not know what else to do. One daughter stated that it really was the only thing she could do to support her mother: "I don't know if there is anything you can say" (26b). Another daughter had similar thoughts about why her support took this form. She recalled being her mother's "sounding board" as she discussed her treatment decisions: "I knew that it was just kind of for her to talk them out and hear them out loud" (36b).

Showing Affection

After their diagnoses, mothers recalled a noticeable increase in the amount of affection they received from their emerging adult daughters. The daughters also recalled that they displayed this form of support more frequently than ever before. Showing affection included giving hugs, saying "I love you," and kissing the mothers. Mothers found this to be atypical of their daughters' behavior. As these daughters were all emerging adults (ages 18–29), it is likely that they were showing this emotional support more so for the first time since adolescence—a time of separation for mothers and daughters.

Mothers found this type of support helpful in their adjustment because it made them feel more "normal" and loved. They also seemed to be appreciative because it was new behavior for their daughters. The mothers frequently noted that the behavior was not "normal," that it was "a lot more frequent than it had been," or indicated that it was "never [done] before." Given that these daughters had just emerged into adulthood and some were even late adolescents when their mother was diagnosed, this increase in affection was likely a striking difference to their mothers. Up until the mother's diagnosis, these relationships were likely characterized by more distance—a dominant feature of mother-daughter bonds when the daughter is in adolescence. One mother indicated how noticeable of a change this was to her:

> She never really gave me a hug or kissed me or said "I love you" before this all happened. Completely changed. She says she loves me all the time, texts me that, gives me a hug now all the time when she sees me. That was not [my daughter]! (28a)

Some daughters also admitted that this type of support was new to them. They felt that they could enact this support after seeing their mothers being affectionate. Other daughters indicated that the diagnosis made them become more "open" to this type of emotional support. Still other daughters mentioned wanting to behave in this way for the "first" time in their relational history. As one daughter said:

> There have been a couple of times where I kind of put my arm on her back, and I would never have done that, I think, before. I never felt the urge to do something like that. . . . I knew she was having trouble. . . . I remember just looking at my mom, making eye contact with her, and putting my arm behind her. (29b)

Mothers also reported valuing this type of support because it became a pattern of communication in their relationship. Their daughters showed this kind of support more consistently by expressing their love every time they said hello or goodbye and each night before they went to bed, or they made sure that it occurred on daily basis. One daughter described her reasoning for consistently displaying affection when engaging in certain interactive activities with her mother:

> Whenever I got off the phone I have to—well, I do not have to say it. It's always like, "Alright—bye—I love you. Alright—bye—I love you. Alright—bye—I love you. Alright—bye—I love you." Put the phone down now! And if you try to leave, it is usually I give her a hug no matter what or where I am going. . . . [What if] something happens? Then you are going to feel bad that you did not give her a hug. So that is always in the back of your mind. (30b)

Being Humorous

Mothers and daughters often made reference to their use of humor to cope with breast cancer. Like those in other dyads, humor was particularly helpful to mothers' adjustment because it made the issue "lighter." As one mother recalled, "We buried a lot of this in funny stuff. . . . You know try to make light of it and try to giggle about it, because that's all you can do" (16a). Moreover, mothers felt that humor served to protect their minds from trauma, help them stay strong, and keep things normal. Although it seemed that mothers often were the source of the behavior, daughters also displayed humor by making jokes, giving their mothers nicknames, and being sarcastic.

Typically, humor helped mothers cope with their "losses." These included the loss of a breast, hair, and menstruation. For instance, daughters often joked with their mothers about being jealous because they did not have to deal with bras, large breasts, or having a period. Daughters also used nicknames for their mothers as their hair grew back (e.g., Chia-Pet). Daughters recalled joking about their mothers' drains after they had a mastectomy (e.g., one daughter called them her mother's grenades), as well as their remaining breast (e.g., Unaboob). One mother shared how her daughter joked with others about why the mother was home from work: "She would tell people this spring, 'Oh no my mom doesn't have cancer! She's just home to be my wedding planner!'" (6a). Another daughter mentioned using a nurse's cap she found from a Goodwill store each time she would give her mother an injection at home to have "fun with it." Daughters often mirrored their mothers' humor as one noted in the following excerpt:

> We were making dinner one day, and my mom goes [to my dad], "Do you want the [mother's name] special?" 'Cause we were having chicken. He's like "What's that?" and she's like, "One breast, two legs. Do you want one?" And I'm like "Mom! Stop!" . . . She's learning to accept it and joke around it. It'll be good stories for later on! (16a)

Staying Positive

Interestingly, diagnosed mothers always felt that daughters' staying positive communication was helpful in their adjustment. This was in contrast to the other groups of dyads, in which this form of emotional support functioned both adaptively and maladaptively. In opposition, mothers diagnosed in midlife felt this support was always adaptive. This difference seemed partly tied to mothers perceiving that the support affected them differently for reasons related to having an emerging-adult daughter. Although mothers felt staying positive made them feel strong and let them know their daughters believed in them, they also observed that positive talk let them know that their daughter was doing okay. This type of support included daughters reassuring their mothers, maintaining a positive outlook or talking positively, encouraging their mothers, and, in a few instances, giving their mothers compliments. Mothers sometimes associated such behavior with their daughters opening up more. As was noted in Chapter 10, these daughters were also typically more avoidant, withdrawn, and distressed over their mothers' diagnosis, and their mothers were understandably more worried for their daughters' well-being. Because of this concerning communication pattern, any positive communication from daughters was likely perceived by these mothers as a good thing.

Many of the diagnosed women described this type of support as important for both mothers' and daughters' well-being. As in the other age groups, sometimes they felt that positivity was a family norm. Yet the mothers really wanted their daughters to have a "positive outlook" regarding their situation. When daughters did act positively, this behavior uplifted their mothers' spirits and made them feel comfortable with how the daughters were coping. As one said:

> She just believed that I had the strength to do this. . . . "Believe. You know, just believe in yourself." And it was like the word in the house. . . . That's what she would tell me. It was almost like it came full circle. It was like what you preach and what you teach comes back. (29a)

Daughters often portrayed this sort of support as having reciprocal effects. Seeing their mothers' strength made them strong and positive.

However, they also admitted that type of support was something they did when at a loss concerning what else to do. They wanted their mothers to be happy. Daughters also seemed to feel a responsibility to be positive because that was how their mothers had behaved with them in the past.

Interestingly, mothers often mentioned enacting positive talk in response to their daughters' communication. For instance, when mothers seemed to be struggling, daughters said encouraging things such as, "You're doing fine," or reassuring their mother with, "It's going to be okay." Mothers frequently reciprocated by saying something like, "I know it's going to be okay. I'm just really tired" or "I'm going to be fine." Mothers seemed to reciprocate or mirror their daughters' positive talk to ensure their daughters they were also okay. Such exchanges seemed to facilitate mothers' adjustment because they otherwise worried about how their daughters were coping.

Staying Normal

It was also especially important to mothers that their daughter enact support that conveyed to them that things were "normal" for them, something that had not been addressed in other age groups. Mothers frequently found this type of emotional support as most helpful in their adjustment. As one mother observed, "I may have discussed this with them, that keeping things normal. . . . There was no reason to change anything because what's best for me [was] . . . for all of us is to go along as we normally are" (26a). Mothers wanted their daughters to maintain their normal routines and to "keep life as normal as possible" (29a). They felt that daughters provided this form of emotional support by sharing with them about their lives, engaging in mundane talk, continuing their lives as usual, maintaining good grades, and acting as if the diagnosis were not all that big a deal. One mother explained how she perceived this as supportive and key to her adjustment:

> I wanted to know what she was doing. . . . Because that made me feel comfortable to know if she was continuing to go, you know, out to lunch with friends or going to her study groups and all that. I wanted to know that she continued on and wasn't sitting there dwelling on me or anything else. . . . For her to continue her life as she is, that's actually, that's comforting to me. That makes me feel the comfort I need to do what I need to do. . . . As long as I know she's doing what she needs to be doing, continuing with her work and her schoolwork, going to go to all her tests, participating in cultural events that she likes. That actually brings me so much comfort. I can sit here and do what I need to do for myself and not be worried about her. I can concentrate on myself more so. . . . For her to be continuing to do that, just like I wanted her to, has been helpful for me. It's been a good thing. (39a)

Daughters also felt that it was important to maintain day-to-day activities, such as watching television together at night, doing their chores on certain days, or, as one daughter put it, continuing to do "the things we would have done together before" (20b). Some daughters noted that "staying normal" served as a distraction from cancer. This was important in preventing their mothers from becoming depressed. In addition, the daughters found that by sharing their lives, they also helped mothers feel needed or, as one daughter stated, "Like she is a big part of our life and like we need her" (28b). Daughters felt this effect uplifted their mothers' spirits and kept their relationship as it was before the diagnosis. One explained:

> That's important to like not focus 100% on the cancer and just like not stopping that part of the relationship. So I think it's important to maintain some sense of normality. I think my mom would have gotten upset or angry if I stopped telling her things just because I didn't want her to have to deal with them or think about them or something, just because she had cancer. (6b)

Similarly, daughters often indicated that *not* staying with their normal routines likely would have been maladaptive. One daughter felt that altering her behavior would have made her mother feel worse. She felt it was important to keep "the normal routine down instead of altering everything and making her feel like 'Everyone's shifting everything around me and I'm such a problem'" (16b).

Being There

"Being there" was an important way in which daughters supported their mothers. Interestingly, however, this form of emotional support was less common in interviews with the current age group of mothers compared with those in other age groups. It is likely that because daughters were either away at school or living in their mothers' houses, "being there" physically was less distinctive as a form of support than in other dyads. Nevertheless, mothers and daughters did mention this as a form of emotional support that always functioned adaptively in their adjustment.

As with the other groups, "being there" referred to the daughters offering to come home, being physically present with their mother, or voicing to the mother that she was "there" for her. When daughters offered to come home, mothers recalled appreciating this support but, at the same time, not wanting it. Typically, mothers explained that they wanted their daughters to stay in school. This reason seemed to connect to the perceived importance of daughters "staying normal." Had daughters come home in the middle of college, their mothers would have been more concerned about them (e.g., falling behind in school, grades suffering, etc.). Daughters seemed to understand their mothers' feelings about them not coming home. When mothers discussed having their daughters physically present, this referred to being present at the hospital for surgery as well as when they shaved their head. Mothers appreciated their daughters' physical presence even more when they experienced especially traumatic aspects of the cancer treatment. Some mothers even recalled surprise visits from their daughters when they were in the hospital or in treatment that was debilitating. Some daughters also mentioned "hanging out" more with their mothers when they were at home to show their mothers they were there for them.

Mothers and daughters also felt that just saying "I am here for you" was helpful in mothers' adjustment. As one mother said:

> Just her verbalizing to me that she's there for me. It's not been doing laundry or anything like that. It's just that she's there and she's concerned and she's there no matter what. Yeah. And I think she appreciates the fact that I've made her a part of it, like taking her to do the wig thing and everything. (8a)

Daughters and mothers felt that in saying this, mothers had a stronger sense of support from their daughters and that they were not alone. One daughter discussed how valuable the support was to her adjustment because it allowed her to provide her mother support more comprehensively:

> It is just being there, letting her know that anything you need or want to talk about, I am here. So just making yourself accessible to her. So I think that was definitely the big thing. Just having her aware that you are there for her because there is not one thing. I do not think there is one thing that you can do as a whole to help the situation. But as long as you, you know, your mom has your support and as long as she knows that, I think that was a big part of, that is what I would say just having her know that I was there and that she had me as a support system. (28b)

"Being there" was helpful in mothers' adjustment because they more strongly felt their daughters' concern for them. By their daughters' being there, their well-being was "boosted." At the same time, daughters appreciated their time with their mothers. It was hard to be away at school during this time when their mothers were trying to cope with such life-altering experiences. They also were aware of how much their mothers wanted to be with them. As one daughter stated, "I mean she is always happy to have more interaction with me, and I felt more—I felt good being around" (39b).

ENACTED EMOTIONAL SUPPORT THAT FUNCTIONS BOTH ADAPTIVELY AND MALADAPTIVELY

The most prominent determinant of whether daughters' behavior could function adaptively or maladaptively related to the daughters' willingness to talk or withdrawal tendencies. Mothers and daughters always seemed to discuss these two forms of behavior in conjunction. Moreover, they were the most prominently mentioned forms of influence in mothers' adjustment to cancer.

Being Willing to Talk Versus Withdrawing

The mothers noted that it was important to them that their daughters show concern by their willingness to talk about their condition. Mothers recalled various signals that daughters were willing to talk about the breast cancer experience, such as calling more frequently or staying in touch more often, particularly during treatment. Mothers interpreted their daughters' calling as more than just "checking in." They felt it showed concern and that they wanted to be a part of their mothers' experiences. This helped mothers to adjust. As one recounted, "She seemed to want to be involved and always asking 'How are you?' . . . I could tell she was concerned and always asking how I was doing and that sort of thing" (26a). At times daughters showed concern by calling and leaving messages if the mothers were not accessible. Other times they made daily phone calls or consistently called after each medical appointment. Mothers found it helpful when their daughters asked questions about how they were feeling.

In daughters enacting this type of support, mothers found themselves more easily able to adjust to cancer in healthy ways. Such supportive behavior let them know that their daughters were willing to talk if they needed to talk. Hence, this enacted support seemed tied to conveying to the mother that their daughter was "there" for them. It was described a bit differently than "being there" support, in that what was most important was that being there in this way meant mothers could talk about their experiences openly. As one mother observed, "I know she's there to talk when I need to talk to her. . . . It's just been the conversation. Just be able to tell her whatever and whenever" (16a). Mothers also felt that daughters' willingness to talk conveyed to them that their daughters cared about them more than before. This growth in their relational intimacy (and maturity in the daughter) was important as one mother in the cohort made clear:

> She seems to be I would say more caring about me. So more sympathetic on her part for me which maybe I hadn't noticed quite as much prior to that. . . . That was a positive thing, where she's more concerned about somebody else. (39a)

Some daughters indicated that being willing to talk was often the only thing they felt they could do to support their mothers because many lived far away from their mothers or were away at college. They felt it was important to allow their mothers to talk about anything they wanted, and they reported that they developed a new appreciation for their mothers, as well as came to realize how important it was to talk to them. Many daughters felt this relational change was a combination of multiple developmental turning points, like their transition to college and becoming an adult, coupled with their mothers' diagnosis. For many daughters, it was hard to separate these as separate turning points. One daughter explained this change in perspective:

> Just kind of a realization that she's not going to be here forever on my part made me want to call her and talk to her more. . . . I think my mom needed me to be there for her and she needed at least one daughter around to be supporting her and things. And I needed to talk to her because I was scared and didn't know what was going to happen. . . . I'll just call her when I'm walking home from class just to say hi and tell her about my day and see how she's doing and stuff like that. And I would never do that before. I would never even think about it. . . . I think it's a combination of the experience and me growing up a little bit. Mostly I think the change is in me than in her. Because I think she always wanted this kind of relationship with me, and I've just never kind of been willing to give it until now. So, yeah, things have changed. (36b)

Mothers felt that when their daughters were willing to talk, they were being more mature. Mothers were happy that their daughters "didn't back away," particularly because they were used to that type of separation or independent behavior from their daughters given that they had just emerged from adolescence. One mother recalled being reassured by such support from both daughters who were entering college:

> At that point when they are getting ready for school and they're not around much and they are kind of pulling away from you a bit. I think that that [daughters calling more] reassured me that she still cared about what was happening with me and that type of thing. And yet if I asked or needed to talk to them or anything, they both were very, very supportive. (26a)

Mothers often perceived this change in their daugh their developmental maturity. Some, like the one belc breast cancer effected this change in her daughter's behavior—rathe, a product of developmental change:

> I think it was her age, you know and thinking six months before—the beginning of that school year, of tenth grade she had a different relationship than maybe we had in January and February. Her maturity and her wanting to talk to me more about things, a willingness to talk to me, I think changed our relationship. So I really don't think it was the diagnosis. (27a)

Regardless of whether mothers felt the changes toward greater willingness to talk were due to daughters' age, the diagnosis, or a combination of the two, they valued them because they revealed that their daughters were "different" now, more open, and becoming more selfless. Daughters also reported that they could now be more open with their mothers. Consequently, mothers felt they adjusted better, and, at the same time, their relationship with their daughters evolved toward greater intimacy.

In opposition were mothers' and daughters' experiences with the daughters' withdrawing. Withdrawal was not uncommon behavior among the daughters. Many of these emerging–adult daughters were in high school (thus, adolescence) when their mothers were diagnosed or just beginning college. They recalled withdrawing from their mother to protect themselves or because they felt talking about it would make their mother's diagnosis an even more distressing reality. Mothers felt daughters withdrew to protect themselves but also because they were still more self-focused as late adolescents or emerging adults.

Daughters signaled this withdrawal by "pushing away" their mothers when they tried to talk to them, "shutting out" their mothers, becoming very quiet, leaving the house, changing the subject, and going to their fathers instead of their mothers. Mothers felt that this behavior functioned maladaptively in their adjustment because it made them feel excluded and unsupported and/or more worried about their daughters' well-being. One mother recalled expecting her 16-year-old daughter to withdraw but not her older daughter, who was a senior in high school. However, when she did, the mother realized that her daughter was still quite young and potentially vulnerable:

> An 18-year-old is very self-centered. And they're supposed to be. And you know in so many ways she's so mature. But in so many ways she's still kind of supposed to be a scared little girl. . . . I was expecting so much with [her] and she was reverting back to being the little girl and

> she was hurt. And you know it all had to do with her age and my expectations and stuff. So there's probably lots of things she could have done that would have supported me a lot more, but I think the biggest problem is that she didn't have the support. She was so scared. She was pushing away every single person: her sister, her boyfriend, to a certain extent her dad. So she didn't have the support either. So that's hard. (16a)

Another mother recalled her daughters withdrawing and not letting her talk. She felt that the withdrawal was for different reasons. More important, however, because her daughters did not let her talk, she felt unsupported:

> I don't think they realize it sometimes, but I think allowing me to talk. I wish sometimes they'd allow me to talk more than they do but they probably don't. . . . The younger one that's more outgoing, she would allow me to talk more if her own life isn't there. But she's interested in her own things. And I don't think she'd see why it was important to talk. But definitely [the other daughter] is not, doesn't want to hear it really. She'll deal with it when she needs to deal with it. (20a)

When mothers had two daughters, they sometimes experienced one daughter withdrawing in their bond and the other daughter not. Some felt that was typical behavior for the daughter who withdrew. Nevertheless, sometimes mothers were surprised and worried about their daughters' behavior. When daughters did not talk or allow their mothers to talk, mothers saw the behavior functioning maladaptively in their adjustment. It made them feel that their daughters were not coping well:

> I think if she talked to me more when I was having surgery would've been helpful because I was really worried about her. Like coming to the hospital. I mean she would just like look at me. I mean I'm sure I looked horrible. But you know just for her to come over and say, "Mom, are you okay?" or "What can I do?" or "How are things going? How are you feeling?" . . . [One daughter] did that. [This daughter] didn't. So I was more worried for her. (28a)

Daughters also recalled that they withdrew and often were unwilling to talk with their mothers. They admitted they would "avoid talking," "get out of the house," "go out and get away from things," and sometimes even tell their mothers they did not want to talk. Upon reflection and once their mothers were in remission, many daughters were remorseful and felt guilty that they had acted this way. As one stated, "I think I probably should have called her more and stuff, and I think if I would have, I think it probably would have helped her" (6bb). Many daughters felt that they mentally could not handle talking to their mothers about their cancer. They perceived withdrawing as the only way they could cope. Many mothers, however, did not feel this behavior was healthy, either for their daughters or them. However, they varied in their approach to handling their daughters' behavior. Some mothers intervened and made their daughters talk. Others sent their daughters to therapists to help them cope. At the same time, some mothers felt it best to let their daughters be. These mothers felt that they would come around in their own time.

14

COPING IN LATER LIFE

Mother-Daughter Dyads

> *[My daughters] always called and I think that was just the biggest support, just knowing that they cared. . . . Just calling more often . . . because it was good just to hear from them. It just meant a lot to hear from them.*
> Diagnosed Later-Life Mother

> *I definitely found myself praising her a lot. I genuinely was impressed by how brave she was. . . . When she lost her hair, she told me she was made 100 times more comfortable about it because I thought she looked really cute and I told her that a lot. . . . I would say, "I like you bald the best. I think it's really cute.". . . If I thought of a compliment, I'd give it to her and I think that made her a lot more comfortable, especially in terms of [her] appearance.*
> Daughter of a Diagnosed Later-Life Mother

As with the midlife-diagnosed mothers, women diagnosed in later life often noted that their daughters' support was always helpful in their ability to adjust to cancer. Rarely did mothers describe their daughters' behavior as not helpful. When they did mention unhelpful forms of support, they typically did so in an indirect manner and seldom described unhelpful interactions in detail, instead focusing more on what their daughters did to help them. Hence, the findings are more heavily focused on adaptive enacted support than maladaptive communication. Collectively, this tendency is in line with developmental research which shows that parents typically describe their relationships with offspring more positively (than do their children), given that a developmental task for parents is to stress continuity and connectedness with children even in adulthood (whereas for children it is to separate and attain independence) (see renowned aging researcher Dr. Vern Bengtson's work on the intergenerational stake hypothesis; Giarrusso, Du, & Bengtson, 2004).

Still, breast cancer was often a meaningful turning point that increased intimacy between these aging mothers and their adult daughters. Daughters prioritized their mothers more, and mothers, in turn, appreciated a newfound effort on the part of their daughters.

ADAPTIVE ENACTED EMOTIONAL SUPPORT

All of these recurrently identified types of support surfaced in interviews involving the other age groups. However, these daughters were also more mature than other cohorts of daughters of diagnosed women, which contributed to mothers and daughters negotiating a more peer-like support system with one another. The nature of this more mature mother-daughter bond is evident in their storied accounts of mutual support for one another.

Being Willing to Listen

As in the younger cohorts, any instance of daughters listening to their mothers talk about their cancer-related experiences and concerns was helpful in mothers' adjustment. Daughters listened to their mothers update them on medical tests and procedures as well as when they began new treatment. As one mother stated, "She listens to everything I have to say" (23a). Mothers often mentioned how consistently their daughters displayed this form of emotional support. One mother felt her daughter was "willing to listen and eager to hear things" (32a).

The importance of daughters' listening to their mothers seemed to be connected to mothers' gratitude for their daughters being patient, understanding, and generous of their time. Mothers were appreciative of their daughters' willingness to listen. Daughters' listening helped in the adjustment to cancer. When asked about what supportive behavior had been most helpful to her, one mother responded:

> I think being able to share what's going on is sort of therapeutic and they [her two daughters] were willing to listen. It wasn't like they didn't have time for me. . . . They just listened patiently. They were understanding. (42a)

Both mothers and daughters also made reference to empathetic listening as helpful in the mothers' adjustment. One mother found this type of listening to be especially important when she shared information with her daughter about the difficult side effects (e.g., mood swings) she experienced from chemotherapy. Unlike the emerging–adult daughters of midlife-diagnosed women who often sympathized by saying "I'm sorry," these daughters' responses were more complex. They responded in a manner that also validated their mothers' feelings. One mother recalled that it was helpful when her daughter responded by saying things such as, "Well, that's really hard" (9a).

Daughters also recognized the importance of listening to their mothers' disclosures. They believed it important to let their mothers talk, empathize, and not interrupt them. As many daughters said, "I just listened." Daughters felt listening was particularly important when mothers were describing side effects from treatment, as well as beginning new ones. As one daughter noted, this type of support helped her mother adjust to the many transitions related to changes in her care:

> It becomes very relevant for her toward the end of treatment and when we're headed into a somewhat unknown time period. . . . Like when we change chemo or when we're about to have surgery or when we were finishing up the post-surgical thing and heading into radiation. All of those things were the unknown. In those particular times, it was really important for her to have somebody, just to be able to say "Okay, this makes me nervous. I'm scared about this. I don't know what I'm thinking here." . . . There's a lot of trepidation. . . . So just listening to her saying "Okay, well, I'm really nervous about this" or whatever. Those times were very important to her. (41b)

As was true of the younger mother-daughter dyads, those in this age group felt that listening was helpful in women's adjustment to cancer. However, they focused more on daughters' listening when mothers talked about procedures and treatment side effects rather than on emotional concerns, a topic in evidence in young-adult-diagnosed daughter-mother dyads' interviews.

Showing Affection

As reported with respect to the younger dyads, showing affection always helped mothers' adjustment to cancer. Women recalled numerous instances when their daughters' affection was both welcome and helpful to them. Although showing affection consisted primarily of daughters giving their mothers hugs, they stressed the importance of other affectionate behavior, including smiling, holding hands, kisses, and engaging in more cuddling or "snuggle time." Some diagnosed mothers recalled that their daughters gave them comforting hugs when they were having "off" days or generally displayed more affection throughout the cancer experience. As one mother observed, "When we're together, we're not afraid to touch each other or hug or hold a hand or something. And that's good" (4a). When daughters showed affection, mothers recalled feeling comforted, loved, reassured, and/or encouraged.

Unlike those in the younger cohorts, several diagnosed mothers also mentioned their daughters' showing affection with respect to their heads after hair loss. Although mention was infrequent with both daughters and their later-life mothers, they saw the value of this behavior as significant. Daughters talked about rubbing their mothers' bald heads often. One mother observed:

> She is always thinking about giving me that extra something—just extra warmth. . . . She just had a way of handling my head nonverbally that was just so loving, reassuring, and fun. That was pretty neat. (9a)

Although middle-adulthood daughters did not undergo chemotherapy (and, hence, did not lose their hair), all of the young-adult daughters did, but they did not report this type of affectionate behavior from their mothers.

Being Humorous

Daughters used humor to support their mothers throughout the cancer transition and portrayed it as something that "gets you through" tough experiences (32a). One mother felt humor was important to her adjustment to cancer because it lightened up dark moments and distressful experiences. A mother described humor functioning adaptively after her mastectomy in this way:

> The girls still laugh about the fact that when I came out of surgery, one of the first things I said to them and I knew that I said it because I can hear myself saying it now was, "She only took one, right?" I looked at

> both of them, and I said, "She only took one off right?" . . . We all have that sense of humor and take life as lightly as you can. You know in a grave situation like this, you just can't dwell on it in that manner. You have to make light of it and just keep going on. (41a)

Daughters seemed to share this perspective with their mothers. As one stated, "If we didn't laugh, sometimes I think we'd just cry all the time" (17b).

Later-life mothers' and their daughters' experiences were similar to those in the previous age group's dyads. Both saw humor as critical to mothers' adjustments because it was instrumental in making cancer-related situations or experiences silly or fun. They mentioned using humor particularly with regard to treatment-related procedures. For instance, one mother described how she and her daughter joked about measuring fluid after surgery because having bags/drains was simply silly looking. Other mothers and daughters made reference to laughing and joking together about treatment side effects, such as nail damage and hair loss. For example, some women used humor to make wig shopping fun. They recalled laughing while trying on outrageous wigs and experimenting with different hair colors and lengths, such as being a "redhead" or "blonde." After hair loss, daughters sometimes gave their mothers funny nicknames such as "Bald Eagle" or "Michael Jordan."

Unlike the younger dyads, the daughters of women diagnosed in later adulthood noted that they had to be careful about their humor. One daughter recalled how she and her sister joked with her mother about getting manicures (after the chemotherapy severely darkened her nails for an extended period of time) and teasing her after she lost her hair and eyebrows from chemotherapy, but in a way that was free of hurt:

> We were routinely making fun of her and razzing her about the fact that she can't draw an eyebrow on to save her life. . . . I'd be looking at her eyebrows, way down below the line of her glasses, and I'm like, "Mom, did you look in the goddamned mirror when you drew that on this morning?" She would just be like, "Oh, shut up! I can't see because I don't have my glasses on!" We made a lot of jokes about very bad eyebrows. . . . She was fairly sensitive about losing her hair, so my sister and I tried to make jokes about that. It was sort of a touchy subject with her, so we tried to make little jokes and pet her little bald head every once in a while, but she was fairly sensitive about that kind of stuff, so we did it a little more lightly on that kind of stuff. . . . I always tried to interject some sort of light-hearted comments so that she would at least chuckle to herself. Sometimes she laughed out loud. . . . I think that was a huge way for her to cope because I forced her into laughing even though she's not really prepared to laugh at that point. (41b)

Lifting Me Up

Like young-adult daughter-mother dyads, those in later-adulthood dyads talked about what they did to cheer up the diagnosed women. This type of emotional support was somewhat different from the younger cohorts, however, in that it primarily consisted of daughters giving or sending their mothers silly or heart-warming cards, flowers, and sometimes gifts, often after surgery and during treatment. Because many daughters lived some distance away, this type of enacted emotional support was especially characteristic of daughters who could not be physically present with their mothers. For instance, daughters sent their mothers sentimental cards expressing how much they meant to them. They also bought their mothers things to help them during treatment, such as yoga equipment or new clothes when they lost weight following chemotherapy. The mothers described instances in which they received gifts from their daughters that were related to their favorite things, hobbies, or interests (e.g., one mother mentioned her daughters buying her a lot of Halloween décor because she loved that holiday).

Sometimes this type of support was frequently in evidence throughout mothers' cancer experience. One daughter recalled supporting her mother in this way. She left her mother small notes around the house throughout her cancer experience: "[I'd] just write like, 'Have a good day! Thinking of you.' Or something like that because I know those things make her smile. So just to make sure to try to cheer her up" (17b). Another daughter made reference to this type of support as a conscious effort on her part to help her mother adjust:

> [I'd] occasionally send a card, having flowers show up at her house, kind of thing. It's just little small things like that. I've always sort of been very aware of how can I put a smile on my mom's face kind of thing. . . . I'll stop by and I'll just leave a quick note at her house. When she gets home she'll see it and she'll laugh. Little things like that. I'm trying to make a conscious effort to do that whenever I can. (41b)

Mothers reportedly found such support uplifting but also motivating. It made them feel that their daughters cared for them and were thinking of them. One mother stressed how important this type of support was when she returned home from the hospital:

> When I got home from the hospital, there were flowers here, and the night before I went to the hospital, [my daughter] bought me this lovely gift then left it here with a card. You know, that was very inspiring. (41a)

As in the case of the younger dyads, efforts to cheer them up were instrumental in keeping diagnosed women's spirits high. However, the actual communicative acts in this age group consisted more of special notes or cards that daughters wrote to their mothers rather than celebratory times together or care packages.

Giving Compliments

Mothers seemed to be especially appreciative when their daughters paid them compliments. Daughters often complimented their mothers about how strong they were, how beautiful they looked, how brave they were, and what wonderful mothers they were to them. This form of communication emerged in other dyads' experiences but primarily in relation to support meant to keep things positive or cheer up the diagnosed women. In this group of dyads' experiences, however, giving compliments most often reflected emotional support mothers received in relation to coping with changes in their physical appearance.

Mothers seemed to value compliments from their daughter about how they looked after their hair loss more than in other types. As one mother stated, "No matter what I looked like, [my daughter would say], 'You know, you are so beautiful'" (32a). Daughters often reassured their mothers that they "looked good" or "beautiful" when they wore scarves, hats, or wigs. For instance, one mother noted how good her daughter's compliments made her feel after she lost her hair: "I mean she was just so sure I looked really cute bald. She didn't think I needed to wear that wig or scarf so she was really complimentary" (9a).

The daughters seemed to understand that their mothers needed to hear these compliments about their appearance, especially during chemotherapy, which included hair loss. One recognized that this aided her mother in adjusting to her new appearance and helped her to feel that she looked okay. This support seemed important in enhancing her mother's self-image and self-esteem:

> She loves when people tell her she looks good, she looks, you know healthy. She loves when people tell her that kind of stuff. That makes her feel really good. So it's just—you know—kind of a—what's the word I'm looking for—a *validation* to her that she seems well, she looks well, you know, those kind of things are important to her. (19b)

Some daughters sensed that their compliments helped their mothers adjust. Other daughters recalled their mothers confirming this. One recalled her mother confirming this directly to her:

> I definitely found myself praising her a lot. I genuinely was impressed by how brave she was and how she was able to, for the most part, really maintain a positive attitude. So I found myself praising that. When she lost her hair, she told me she was made 100 times more comfortable about it because I thought she looked really cute and I told her that a lot. And when she would come see me, I would say, "I like you bald the best. I think it's really cute." . . . If I thought of a compliment, I'd give it to her and I think that made her a lot more comfortable, especially in terms of appearance things. Once she was losing her hair, she was initially really nervous and self-conscious about it. (9b)

The importance of compliments for later-life women related most directly to their feelings concerning hair loss. These women were self-conscious about their appearance because of this side effect, and their daughters were aware of their mothers' struggles with this aspect of the cancer experience. Although other women, particularly those in young adulthood, experienced hair loss from chemotherapy, this was the first group of dyads to note the significance of receiving compliments in helping them cope with this difficult physical change.

Being There

Like those in the middle-adulthood daughter-mother dyads, later-adulthood-diagnosed mothers often indicated that their daughters' presence or "being there" was helpful in their adjustment to cancer. Unlike young-adult dyads (and like midlife dyads), these women perceived this type of support as always adaptive. They frequently characterized this type of emotional support as "just being there," "knowing that she was there," or her "physical presence." Mothers appreciated their daughters enacting this type of emotional support in such cases as being with them for appointments, shopping for wigs, celebrating events, and helping at home. Many of the mothers also noted that they wanted their daughters' company. They felt that by her "just being there" or by "knowing she was there," they were more at peace. Additionally, daughters keeping their mothers company gave them a sense that they were not alone and that they could rely or count on their daughters for support. This increased their comfort level. One mother recalled how her daughter came home to be with her:

> She dropped everything she was doing and came home, which I didn't anticipate her doing that, but it was great for me. You know, she gave up everything. . . . She gave things up. And she was there all the way. I mean she came home and actually lived here. So she was right with me the whole way. Very positive influence. I mean I was glad she was here 'cause, you know, you do need that. (4a)

"Being there" was especially important in helping mothers adjust to hair loss. One mother recalled her daughter being with her when she shopped for wigs, lost her hair, adjusted to wearing the wig, and adjusted to taking the wig off once her hair began to come in. She stated, "I rely on her to be involved in that way" (19a). Daughters also frequently indicated that "being there" was the best thing they could do to help their mothers adjust. One even had moved home shortly before her mother's diagnosis:

> It's very weird, but I think it was a good thing that I moved home when I did, before that happened to her. . . . With me being back home with her is probably the best thing I could've done. Because otherwise I wouldn't have been living with her and I couldn't, you know, just be her sounding board or whatever she wanted me to be if I wasn't here all the time. So I think that was probably the best thing. . . . I think I needed her as much as she needed me to be there. Just that I knew she'd be okay. (17b)

As this daughter explained, "being there" for their mothers not only helped their mothers adjust, but it also helped daughters cope themselves. One daughter noted the importance of this sort of emotional support when accompanying her mother to her treatment appointments, both for her mother and herself:

> There's a huge level of emotional support just being able to go there. . . . There's a huge emotional draw for me to be there supporting her because I know that that level of support, number one, she's only going to get from me. And number two, she definitely counts on it. I wouldn't have it any other way. I wouldn't have not been there to support her. (41b)

ENACTED SUPPORT THAT FUNCTIONS BOTH ADAPTIVELY AND MALADAPTIVELY

Although mothers in this cohort tended to concentrate on how helpful their daughters' support was to their adjustment to cancer, at times they did lightly discuss unhelpful support that proved to be maladaptive. Some of these categories of supportive behavior (*staying normal* and *staying positive*) reflect emotional support communication enacted in the younger dyads although described and functioning differently. These women also identified new forms of support specific to this phase of the mother-daughter relational life span and how breast cancer functioned as a turning point that increased intimacy in their bond. In particular, it was important to mothers that they perceived their daughters making an effort and offering suggestions.

Making an Effort

This first type of supportive communication addressed a notable change that mothers witnessed in their daughters' communicative behavior—a change that showed new communicative and relational sides to the daughter. Mothers frequently described two similar changes in communicative behavior that were also ways daughters emotionally supported them. They consistently discussed these in relation to their recognition that their daughters were making an effort to help them adjust. The communication pattern required two subcategories to capture the two similar but distinct communicative changes that mothers felt daughters made in supporting them: *spending more time together* and *calling/talking more*. These were not only important to mothers' adjustment but also in redefining the nature of their mother-daughter bond.

Spending More Time Together

It was important to mothers that their daughters make an effort to spend time together. Daughters often talked about wanting to be around their mothers more and taking corresponding steps to do so. Daughters described this motivation in relation to a newfound understanding that their time together could be limited. As one daughter stated, "We have created a new sense of we really need to be together as much as we can. . . . Whereas maybe before, it was sort of taken for granted" (41b). Daughters who lived at a long distance attempted to spend as much time with their mothers as they could. One daughter reported making a few surprise long-distance visits to see her mother after the diagnosis and throughout treatment:

> I think there was a big realization of what we had and how special it was. . . . I really made an effort to get home or to have plans for her to come to [my home]. . . . It was just really hard for me not to be there. (9b)

The adaptive nature and importance of this communication to later-life mothers specifically focused on the meaning of daughters' *effort* versus her actual physical presence or companionship. Mothers receiving this type of enacted support always discussed it in relation to noticing how much of an effort their daughters made to see them more often. Mothers recognized that before the diagnosis, daughters chose to spend more time with their own children, families, or friends rather than with them. It was their daughters' extra effort (or being "careful" to be coming home) that was critical to mothers' estimation of the value of this type of communicative support. One mother described this change in her daughter, saying:

> My daughters didn't always come to see [me]. The kids are in school or there was always a reason. . . . We were visiting them more often. But once I was diagnosed, they all made an effort to come and see me. (12a)

Many of the diagnosed women in this age group felt that by coming home more and making time to be together, daughters were helping them adjust to the cancer. One mother stressed how important this was to her:

> I feel we try to do as much together, and it's obvious when she comes home that she likes to make sure she spends time with me. I don't think that would happen otherwise. She'd be in her busy way, which is nice. (4a)

When mothers explained why they felt this behavior was supportive and helpful, they uniformly referred to how important their daughters' effort was rather than how they spent their time together, their daughter's presence, or having companionship. This type of communication may have been especially important to these mothers as all but one daughter was in emerging or young adulthood. Thus, they were closer to the developmental period in which daughters tend to separate from their mothers and spend more time with peers.

Daughters made an effort to see their mothers and spend time together in such ways as stopping by the mothers' house unexpectedly, making surprise long-distance visits, arranging mother-daughter activities (e.g., going to the spa, watching *Sex and the City*, candle-making), taking trips together, spontaneously going shopping together, arranging larger family shared time or activities (e.g., planning a cookout or picnic), and bringing over grandchildren (i.e., the daughters' children). Not all of daughters' enacted support in spending time with their mothers related to cancer (e.g., treatment and appointments). Hence, this type of support again differed from "being there" as their shared time was not health-specific. Mothers perceived this form of emotional support as daughters wanting to spend time with them—something that conveyed to them their daughters' love and appreciation. This was not about "being there" as a supportive presence in the health setting, caregiver, cancer partner, or companion, but instead efforts to enhance mothers' emotional well-being in general.

Daughters often mentioned making an effort to spend time together to boost their mothers' emotions on down days, to ensure they were not lonely, to engage them in fun activities, to make sure they were staying busy (i.e., as a distraction), and to make sure they felt loved. One daughter recalled her mother sharing time together when she did not feel well. When she asked her mother what she needed, she always replied that she wanted a visit from her and/or with the grandkids:

> I just try [when] I know she's feeling down, I'll just get her out shopping. I'll take the kids down. They always seem to, you know, make her laugh. . . . We'll just go do something just to perk her up. . . . I take her out to lunch a lot or to the mall . . . just to get her thinking about other things. And usually, that does the trick, . . . you know, keeping her busy with the grandkids, keep getting her away from the house, anything that's getting her out of her environment and, you know, just distracting her. (19b)

This type of support had reciprocal adaptive effects. Daughters admitted that by spending more time together, they could make sure their mother was doing okay, which in turn brought them comfort.

This form of support typically always functioned adaptively. The only instance in which mothers referred to it as maladaptive was to say that they wanted more of it. They would have liked to have had more time with their daughters. Doing so would have been even more helpful to their adjustment to cancer, as one mother said: "I think I would have liked to have seen them [her daughters] more, but you know that wasn't even possible either way. To me that would have been more helpful" (12a). Like this mother, others were understanding of daughters' limitations in being able to visit all the time as daughters often had children themselves, worked full time, or lived a notable geographic distance away. Interestingly, daughters often wished they could spend more time with their mothers throughout this experience. Many mentioned how hard it was not to be together.

Calling/Talking More

Mothers and daughters reported talking more with one another throughout the cancer experience. However, again, like "spending more time together," mothers characterized this support as helpful in relation to daughters making a notable effort to talk to their mothers frequently. Often the support consisted of daughters calling more to check in on their mothers to see how they were doing. The calling was sometimes associated with how mothers were feeling after cancer treatment and appointments. For mothers, it was their daughters' effort that was important to them in their adjustment because it made them feel that their daughters cared, were concerned about them, and were interested in their well-being. Mothers also felt that this type of enacted support was helpful because they wanted to hear from their daughters.

The mothers spoke of this support as the daughters' initiative to stay in touch. Some found this was "bizarre," as it was not typical of their daughter. Nonetheless, these women felt this support was instrumental in their adjustment. One said,

> They always called, and I think that was just the biggest support, just knowing that they cared. . . . Just calling more often . . . because it was good just to hear from them. It just meant a lot to hear from them. (12a)

Like the young-adult daughters of midlife-diagnosed mothers, daughters in the current age group wanted to talk with their mothers more. One daughter volunteered, "I would feel bad if I didn't talk to her for the day" (32b). Daughters admitted that they consciously called and talked with their mothers with greater frequency, often to check in on them. When daughters were at a long distance, this enacted support seemed particularly helpful for both mothers and daughters. As one daughter recalled:

> I [was] making it an important part of my day, making that a priority to know what's going on with her. Whereas before, even though we're really close, I may have just checked on her a couple times a week . . . it's become total priority for me to know what's going on with her at this point. (41b)

Interestingly, these communicative acts are similar to previous dyads' experiences with "mothering," as well as "being willing to talk." Yet the mothers did not refer to this behavior in a maternal way. Moreover, mothers did not discuss daughters' calling in relation to their willingness to talk. Instead, women related calling/talking more to their daughters' making an effort to stay in touch—an effort that they found previously uncharacteristic of their daughters' behavior. Although this type of emotionally supportive communication could be conceived as mutual mothering or mothering support, neither mothers nor daughters described it in those terms. Moreover, a notable characteristic of mothering support illustrated by diagnosed daughters and their mothers was its maladaptive properties such that this communication often became overbearing. In contrast, later-adulthood mothers never mentioned feeling that their daughters were overdoing it or becoming overbearing when discussing their efforts to calling and staying in touch.

The only instance in which mothers referred to this type of support as maladaptive related to daughters not believing them. This sometimes occurred when daughters called to check in on how their mothers were doing. Mothers said that they were fine, but their daughters did not always believe them. For mothers, it was important that their daughters trust what they said and not question them in a manner that conveyed distrust. For instance, one mother said,

> I liked that fact that she cared and wanted to know things. Sometimes when I would just say things, she'd say, "Well, are you sure?" and I would say, "Yeah." That was the annoying [thing] that [she] believe me that I was okay and everything. (32a)

Staying Normal

Many women recalled that the most helpful thing their daughters did was "keeping things normal." Like midlife-diagnosed mothers, later-life-diagnosed mothers felt that certain communicative acts were key in conveying to them that life remained normal. This support was important to mothers' adjustment because they did not want their condition to transform their daughters' (or their) lives. They did realize that cancer inevitably altered their lives. Nonetheless, it was still important to them that their daughters act as normally as possible because that led them to feel that everything was okay. Pertinent communication included sharing their personal lives with their mother, engaging in mundane talk, and not showing any emotion in their mothers' presence about the diagnosis.

Mothers wanted their daughters to share with them details about their personal lives and to learn about their daily activities, as well as their grandchildren's well-being. By hearing about their daughters' lives, the mothers reportedly adjusted better. At times this behavior helped because it made mothers still feel needed as a mom. As one mother explained:

> It made me feel like she needed me as a mom. . . . That gave me a reason to live. It gave me another reason, something to hold on to, to keep me going and I felt like I was needed. (12a)

Similar to midlife mothers, these mothers also noted that when daughters shared details of their lives with them, they worried less about how they were coping. Hearing about their lives helped mothers feel that their daughters were doing well, which therefore lessened their distress and worry for their daughters. This form of emotional support also kept mothers from thinking about their condition constantly. In effect, this type of support made things feel more normal.

When daughters recognized their mothers' desire for this support, they were willing to talk about their own lives more often. However, they often mentioned struggling with whether to engage in this type of communication. Some daughters, at first, did not perceive that staying normal in this way could function supportively. This may have been more of an issue for daughters still in emerging adulthood. One daughter described the dilemma:

> At first my reaction was definitely oh, I don't want to be a burden. I don't want to load her with little things that are bothering me. That was only for probably a month or so after the diagnosis and after that, I realized she actually liked hearing about all of that stuff and helping me figure it out. . . . She really enjoys being a part of my life. . . . That means not just hearing about all the good things that I was doing but hearing about the stress and the crazy times too. (9b)

Some mothers also perceived engaging in mundane everyday talk with their daughters as supportive. They considered it emotionally supportive because it provided a distraction from cancer and made them feel that life was still normal. One mother described this enacted support functioning adaptively in this way:

> We would talk every day and talk about things and people and you know, what was going on. So yeah, this does take your mind off of it and just keeps you more involved in everyday life you know, in getting through. So that's—I think that's good because you don't want to dwell on it too much. . . . You know I found that if you are just home and by yourself, you would think of it [cancer] constantly. (32a)

Finally, mothers stated that not seeing their daughters become emotional about their cancer kept life nearly normal. Many women felt that by not showing emotion, ironically, daughters emotionally supported them. Some mothers even told their daughters not to cry in front of them. This reportedly functioned adaptively, in that it helped them worry less about how their daughters were coping. In not seeing their emotion, mothers believed their daughters were handling it okay. Such mothers explained that if their daughters were to show distress about the diagnosis, it would "break" them or make them worry. Some mothers recognized that, although their daughters withheld emotion in front of them, they may not have done so in their own personal time or when talking with their spouses, fathers, sisters, or friends. Diagnosed women in other age groups also mentioned not wanting to see their mothers'/daughters' emotion. However, these women also did not discuss this in relation to keeping things normal.

Interestingly, not showing emotion and talking about the daughters' personal lives could also function maladaptively. Although mothers did not heavily focus on this, some did briefly mention it. For instance, one mother felt that she did not want her daughter to share her problems with her because she would, in fact, feel burdened. However, this particular mother and daughter were dealing with more serious, long-term problems in the daughter's life (e.g., problematic behaviors such as addiction or reckless behavior) rather than day-to-day stresses. Hence, the intensity of the daughter's problems likely affected whether such disclosures were helpful to mothers' adjustment.

Additionally, although most mothers reported not wanting to see their daughters' negative emotional reactions to the disease, one mother offered a different perspective:

> I didn't want her more upset than me, you know. The fact that you worry about your daughter when you are like going through this. . . . You worry about the effects [of this on her]. . . . But it's funny. I mean if they weren't upset you felt like they didn't care. . . . I think a little bit you needed to know that this affected [her]. (32a)

Offering Suggestions

Women in this cohort also were appreciative of daughters' suggestions they felt were helpful in positively enhancing their adjustment to cancer. This type of emotional support had rarely been mentioned by other cohorts. Suggestions related to treatment side effects, finding new clothes during treatment, buying and styling wigs, styling hair after chemotherapy, and how to stay active during treatment (e.g., taking walks and doing yoga). This type of support seemed to be most helpful to mothers when they perceived it as encouraging or insightful. Often the suggestions were primarily informational in nature. However, mothers more frequently discussed this form of support in relation to helping them feel better.

Suggestions frequently addressed mothers' adjustment to their new hair growth after chemotherapy. One mother talked about her daughter helping her in this way once her hair began to grow back after chemotherapy treatment ended:

> She was the one who encouraged me to go with this shorter hair style. And she was the one who would get to the point: "Okay, Mom. It's time to take the wig off. You got a little bit of hair. That's as good as style!" And so forth and so on. I mean, these [comments] are what I mean. She's so encouraging. . . . And so we went to this girl. I couldn't quite explain what to do because I have always had long hair. (9a)

Mothers also seemed to feel that their daughters' suggestions were helpful when they perceived their daughters had specialized knowledge about a particular issue, particularly during interactions about side effects. One mother recalled not being able to drink water after her taste buds changed. She expressed her concern to her daughter about staying hydrated. Her daughter, who was active in sports, suggested various sports drinks for her mother to try, which the mother perceived as especially helpful. Another mother talked about her experiences with various medications her daughter also had taken at one time. She described to her daughter the related side effects of these medications (e.g., tingling sensation in the legs) and noted how valuable her daughter's suggestions were in helping her manage the uncomfortable effects.

The only circumstance in which this type of enacted support seemed not to function adaptively was when the suggestions concerned hair loss. Women diagnosed in later adulthood were particularly self-conscious of their appearance after losing their hair during chemotherapy. Both mothers and daughters talked about the trauma associated with this loss, as well as the drastic manner in which mothers' hair fell out (e.g., in clumps). To help mothers cope, daughters often suggested they shave their hair off once they began to lose it rather than watch it all fall out. However, this was not a suggestion that many mothers received well. Once women lost their hair or when their hair started to grow back, daughters often suggested to their mothers that they not wear their wigs. Again, mothers seemed particularly sensitive and resistant to such suggestions. One daughter discussed her experience with this:

> My sister and I both tried to get her to shave her head and go bald, and she flipped out about that. We didn't really visit that a lot. . . . Once her hair starting growing back in, then it became the kind of thing where we continued. "Okay, you hair is growing in. It looks cute. It's a really short hair style. You should turf the wig." She wasn't comfortable and would get pissed off and irritated with us continuing to bother her, so we just let it go. (41b)

In the previous examples of daughters' emotional support in the form of compliments, it was evident that mothers diagnosed in later adulthood were especially challenged in adjusting to hair loss. Mothers' experiences with daughters' suggestions further demonstrate that this physical change is an especially difficult one for later-life mothers to adjust to. As such, daughters' suggestions about how mothers wear their hair needed to be carefully communicated if they were to be perceived as helpful. It is likely that this experience is tied to a mother's need for privacy, as was illustrated in Chapter 11. Later-life-diagnosed women often described wearing wigs as a means of keeping their illness private.

Staying Positive

In line with most of the other cohorts of dyads, mothers in later adulthood felt that daughters talking to them positively helped them adjust in a healthy manner. Staying positive involved daughters reassuring their mothers about cancer-related distresses they shared, encouraging them to keep fighting the disease, and making sure that an upbeat outlook had high priority during difficult times. Mothers felt that this type of enacted communication was most helpful in making them feel better, particularly on down days, and in motivating them to stay strong and beat cancer. For instance, mothers referred to daughters' positive communication in such terms as it "picks me up," makes one "upbeat," or "makes me feel better." They also felt this behavior motivated them to persist. In the words of one mother,

> She'll just tell me to think positively. If I say something negative, she says, "No, you can't say that." You know, "I don't want to hear that." But in a good way—not a bad way. She's a positive motivator. . . . She's very in tune to how I feel. Picks me up, you know? (4a)

Many mothers indicated that they could not recall an instance in which their daughters were not positive with them. These women also seemed to feel that it was important for them to remain positive for their daughters' well-being, as well as the rest of the family's. Several mothers saw this behavior as stemming from a view of life they used to help each other adjust. One mother characterized the reciprocal nature of this enacted support with her daughter and the rest of her family in the following way: "I was positive about it. That made them feel positive about it. Or maybe I felt so positive about it because they talk positively about it" (43a).

Daughters often discussed providing support for their mothers by talking positively to them. For instance, one daughter mentioned reading from a daily affirmation book with her mother. She felt that this form of positive interactive activity was instrumental to their adjustment: "It kind of helped us wake up and at least think, 'Okay! Today's going to be better'" (17b). Daughters also talked about reassuring their mothers that they were "doing so well." Many women tried to reframe the situation and help their mothers see that "things could be worse." Several daughters felt that this type of support was helpful in motivating their mothers to remain strong. For instance, one said,

> I think that when something like this happens, if you're not positive everybody suffers. You know, like the person who has it suffers because you're not really supporting them because all you're doing is

> talking negative. You know? That doesn't make them feel better, and it makes them feel worse about themselves. If you're positive, they have a better outlook on it, like, "Okay—You're right. I am almost done [with treatment]." You know? They want to get it done. They want to get it done, and they want to be fine when it's done. (32b)

Some daughters admitted that they felt their mothers were struggling with extreme sadness and depression and that the positive talk was the only way to help them manage their emotional distress.

Although mothers rarely talked about this behavior as anything but helpful, some did refer to times when their daughters used positive communication to prevent them from speaking negatively. These women felt that their daughters would not allow them to talk about their cancer in any way but positively. One mother asserted that "negative talk" was just not in her daughter's vocabulary. Although mothers seemed to appreciate the consistency of their daughters' positive nature, some women also talked about wanting to just vent. According to one mother,

> If someone would ask me how I felt or whatever and if I would talk about it in a negative way, she would not be happy about that. She wants that positive attitude. She would say, "Don't dwell on the negative." She still tells me if I start being negative. (19a)

When asked whether she felt as if she still wanted to talk (negatively), the mother replied affirmatively but nevertheless defended her daughter's behavior:

> Yeah, I think so. Let me get it out of my system, kind of thing. [But] She is just being positive.

Other mothers felt their daughters' positive talk sometimes blocked their ability to vent. Similar to those in other age groups, these diagnosed women perceived that positive communication was not always helpful. However, these women described this in relation to having their communication censored, as opposed to not having their feelings validated (young- and middle-adult daughters' experiences). Hence, for later-adult-diagnosed mothers, daughters' positive talk did not help them adjust when it prevented them from having an outlet to just vent or expel their distress.

Table 14.1 Mothers' and Daughters' Enacted Emotional Support

In this type of mother-daughter bond	*these forms of emotional support always functioned adaptively*	*whereas the following forms of emotional support functioned both adaptively and maladaptively depending upon contextual factors*
young-adulthood diagnosed daughter-mother bonds	being willing to listen showing affection being humorous lifting me up	being there mothering staying positive validating decisions
middle-adulthood diagnosed daughter-mother bonds	being willing to listen being humorous being there	mothering staying positive
middle-adulthood diagnosed mother-daughter bonds	being willing to listen showing affection being humorous staying normal staying positive being there	being willing to talk versus withdrawing
later-adulthood diagnosed mother-daughter bonds	being willing to listen showing affection being humorous lifting me up giving compliments being there	making an effort spending time together talking/calling more staying normal offering suggestions staying positive

Part VII

JOURNALING MOTHER–DAUGHTER COMMUNICATION DURING TREATMENT

Triangulated Findings

Parts V and VI provided vivid depictions using mothers' and daughters' storied accounts of how they coped together through openness, avoidance, and emotional support behavior. These communicative experiences can contribute to enhancing women's coping and adjustment to the disease, thereby improving their well-being, or work against their ability to cope in healthy ways. These women's shared, authentic mother-daughter stories help bring to the forefront the many factors (e.g., such as age or developmental maturity, the breast cancer issue at hand, the relational role of the diagnosed woman) that can contribute to whether openness, avoidance, and emotional support function adaptively or maladaptively.

Part VII further explores the potential adaptive nature of mother-daughter communication by examining the nature of these behaviors when coping during a particularly challenging phase of the cancer trajectory: when women undergo cancer treatment of radiation or chemotherapy. Each chapter in Part VII represents a mother-daughter pair diagnosed in a particular age group. Thus, a mother-daughter story is presented as a portrayal of coping during each phase of the life span: young, middle, and later adulthood. Their stories depict the nature of the behavior previously presented (mother-daughter openness, avoidance, and emotional support) but in situ, or within the environment they occurred and, specifically, during treatment, a prominent and often more challenging phase of the cancer experience.

The reports include the analysis of diaries and diary interviews and follow Creswell's (2007) 33-33-33 pattern of organization: description of the setting (narrative information pertaining to contextual background), themes (patterns of mother-daughter openness, avoidance, and emotional support according to their accounts), and interpretation of the analysis in conjunction with findings from the interviews. Pseudonyms for the diary authors appear in place of actual women's names to ensure confidentiality.

The diary case studies also serve as a validation tool or a means to validate study results using additional methods to determine whether the same findings emerge. The data from the diaries and diary interviews were compared with findings from the in-depth interviews to enrich our understanding of how mother-daughter communication impacts the breast cancer coping experience. As previously noted, one case study is presented or represents each developmental period in which women are diagnosed. However, two cases are presented for later-life-diagnosed women's mother-daughter dyads given that their daughters varied more in age (often a 10-year gap), and typically daughters were either emerging or young adults. This was done to account for variations in coping experiences due to daughters being in different developmental periods of life.

At times women's mother-daughter communication noted in diaries during treatment differed somewhat from women's narrative interviews. At other times the diaries were congruent with the interview findings. Because both mother and daughter were journaling about their shared experiences at the same time, the interactive nature of mother-daughter coping also comes to the forefront. In addition, these interactions further depict the interconnected nature of open, avoidant, and emotional support communication as the women negotiate coping together. Table 18.1 is presented at the end of Part VII to provide a visual comparison of findings triangulated from data collected via interviews, diaries, and diary interviews.

15

A PORTRAYAL OF COPING DURING YOUNG ADULTHOOD AS A DAUGHTER

Ana is 36 years old and self-described as happily married. She and her husband have three young children. She works as a registered nurse and is completing an online graduate program. Both of her parents are living and married. She has a younger sister, whom she refers to as her "best friend." Her parents and sister live a few hours away.

Ana was first diagnosed with stage II breast cancer at the age of 33. Nearly three years later, she was told she had a recurrence. The cancer had advanced to stage IV. At the time of her first diagnosis, Ana underwent a bilateral mastectomy, reconstruction, and chemotherapy for about four months. She also tested positive for a breast cancer gene and, in an effort to prevent a recurrence, had her ovaries removed. After the second diagnosis, she underwent three months of traditional chemotherapy and, thus, lost her hair for the second time. At the time of this study, she was in a clinical trial with another chemotherapy drug receiving treatment for three straight weeks followed by one week off. She had been told that there was no end date for the treatment and that it would remain continuous.

Lily is Ana's mother. She is 58 years old and feels very close to Ana, as well as her other daughter. Lily struggles with anxiety. She has managed anxiety-related mental wellness concerns for years and felt her anxiety may have increased since her daughter was diagnosed. Lily disclosed that she sometimes feels very alone in her concern for Ana. She perceives that her husband (Ana's father) is not very supportive of her but does not want to burden Ana with her concerns. She often seeks her other daughter's support to cope with her anxiety. She feels close to Ana and believes she "knew" something was wrong even before she was diagnosed both times. During Ana's recovery from the first diagnosis, Lily came and stayed with her for a while. Ana found her mother to be very helpful in assisting her with caring for her young children.

Lily and Ana have a close relationship that is not without difficulties. They talk via telephone every day and update each other on how they are doing and their daily schedule. These conversations usually consist of mundane, everyday chatter. Ana describes her mother as "always there" and caring but notes that she can sometimes be overbearing. She often seeks her sister's support during such times. However, Ana did disclose that since her diagnosis, little things her mother did that used to bother her now affect her much less.

During the two weeks that Ana and Lily kept diaries, communication between them was long distance. The conversations ranged from 5 to 20 minutes, with most calls lasting about 10 minutes. Although both women initiated calls, most of the time Ana would return her mother's call when she had some time to talk. Ana wrote about 10 interactions, and Lily wrote about 12. Only Lily wrote entries (10) in which she mentioned thinking about cancer or cancer-related experiences that she did not share with her daughter for various reasons. Lily's diary entries were in-depth and extensive whereas Ana typically only wrote a sentence or two. Only Ana participated in a diary interview once both women had completed their 2-week diaries.

OPENNESS DURING TREATMENT: DISCLOSED TOPICS AND REASONS FOR OPENNESS

Most of Ana and Lily's conversations were general updates of how each other was doing and what their plans entailed. Ana's talk focused mostly on updating her mother concerning how her children were doing and what activities they were engaged in. For instance, Ana was busy planning a birthday party for one of her children. She also shared with her mother her graduate school-related stress (e.g., writing a paper about her cancer experience).

Although their talk was mostly mundane conversation, Ana did talk openly with her mother about a few cancer-related topics. Specifically, she communicated about her concerns regarding *medical decisions* as well as *diagnostic testing and results.* She told her mother about her uncertainty about when to get a flu shot—that she was nervous about having a flu shot when she also had a cold and allergies due to the poor weather. She also was further concerned she might receive negative results from an upcoming bone scan. When she received the test results, she shared them with her mother.

Ana also openly shared with her mother about some *treatment side effects* she recently encountered. For instance, she talked about her hair and eyebrows growing in (which she had lost during traditional chemotherapy). Ana also disclosed more emotional side effects. She shared with her mother that she was feeling fatigued. She went further in her disclosure in noting that she felt there was just too much going on in her life. She told her mother that she felt that she just wanted to take a day off and "chill." Lily wrote about her concerns in her diary that Ana was "working too hard. . . . I just don't want her to take on too much." However, Lily also felt that, at times, being busy was helpful to Ana's adjustment to cancer because it "keeps her mind busy."

In her diary, Lily noted that she was waiting for Ana to bring up issues related to cancer because she did not want to express her concern. In commenting about this, she wrote, "Why borrow trouble?" Lily also agonized over all that her daughter had to worry about at such a young age. She seemed to be aware of her daughter's need to discuss her worries. Yet she also seemed to appreciate her daughter's need to talk with other individuals. After giving her daughter advice about the flu shot, she wrote, "So many anxious things for her to worry about at 36. I felt better because she was going to her breast cancer support meeting."

Ana indicated that her reason for talking about these matters was to *share good news* (about test results), as well as to *seek her mother's support.* For instance, Ana felt that it was important to tell her mother about good test results because it was "sharing good news" together. This reason tied to her desire to *protect her mother* from worry. When asked in the diary interview why she shared the test results with her mother, she responded:

> It was probably me [wanting to spread] the good news. . . . And I know she worries so I was calling to let her be relieved and not be tensed up thinking, "Oh my gosh, oh my gosh! How's her results?" So it was kind of like for both of us in a sense.

Ana further explained that she openly communicated about these issues because she values her mother's opinion. She wanted her support. Specifically, she wanted her mother's reassurance that her future test results would be okay. Ana shared her feelings about why she freely shared her thoughts on upcoming diagnostic testing:

> I was really nervous about the bone scan. . . . I always go, "Mom, do you have any bad feelings?" She's pretty on the money with that stuff. You know it's just like a mother's intuition. She's like, "Honey, I think everything is gonna be fine. Don't worry." And that just kind of like gives me that little reassurance that okay. She thinks everything is okay, and even if she is lying to me, it gave me that all sense of hope that I didn't worry as much. . . . That kind of soothes me in a sense because she's okay with it.

This experience highlights the interactive nature of open communication and emotional support. As Ana discloses her concerns about test results to seek support, Lily offers Ana reassurance by staying positive and saying everything will be okay. The interview findings showed that seeking support was one reason that young-adult women diagnosed with breast cancer disclosed their cancer-related experiences to their mothers. However, the diary and diary interview reveal the importance of this interdependent dynamic between openness and emotional support communication.

The results of the diary and diary interview mirror the findings from the interviews in that Ana's openness was more medically focused and, yet, at times she addressed her emotions. The reasons for openness also matched. Ana was open as a means of seeking support. However, a new reason for open communication emerged: *to share good news*. This motive for openness may be particularly critical when women are in treatment. During this phase of cancer, women frequently receive a multitude of tests to assess the efficacy of the treatment in fighting the disease. It is particularly important to hear that the treatment is working because it likely influences the women's future outlook of survival. Sharing good news may be even more heightened given that Ana was dealing with a recurrence and continuous treatment. It is also important to note that mundane talk was a much more prominent feature of their mother-daughter talk. Although women were to include references to non-cancer-related talk in their diaries, Ana and Lily seemed to keep their conversations sharply focused on their daily issues rather than Ana's cancer. This communication pattern may be linked to another form of support noted in other age groups of dyad's interviews: *keeping things normal*.

AVOIDANCE DURING TREATMENT: AVOIDED TOPICS AND REASONS FOR AVOIDANCE

Ana admitted that the only matters she strenuously avoided in interactions with her mother were her mother's problems, concerns, or complaints. She avoided talk about these altogether and changed the subject when her mother brought up any complaints. Ana stated that her reason for avoiding such talk was that she found it too *distressful*. She admitted feeling stressed when her mother talked about her own personal worries, gripes, or concerns. Her motive for avoiding such discussions was likely to *protect herself*. However, Ana also stated that she was really trying to respect the possibility that her mother might need support too and, therefore, to be more understanding and reflective of her positive features.

Ana's diary and diary interview revealed that she avoided *distressful topics*. She was motivated to avoid this communication to *protect herself*. Again, these findings validate patterns of communication that emerged in the interview data. Young-adult daughters noted that they avoided topics they perceived as uncomfortable or distressing in an effort to protect themselves from unnecessary angst. Interestingly, Lily felt that she avoided disclosing her personal concerns quite often. As previously noted, she had 10 entries in which she wrote about distresses she did not share with Ana and often mentioned disclosing to other people (e.g., her other daughter as well as her own mother) about these matters. She admitted that sometimes she needed to hear that "everything would be okay." Due to Lily's self-described heightened anxiety, she may have voiced more distresses to Ana than she typically would when feeling less anxious. Ana and Lily jointly described Lily as a pessimist, so this behavior may have been somewhat commonplace in their relational history. Regardless, this finding indicates that this mother-daughter communication dynamic is not necessarily helpful in Ana's adjustment to cancer. Thus, her avoidance of distressful topics likely functioned adaptively in her adjustment to the disease.

ENACTED EMOTIONAL SUPPORT DURING TREATMENT

Lily enacted various types of emotionally supportive communicative behaviors with her daughter during treatment: *being humorous*, *staying positive* (reassurance, sharing survivor's stories), *validating decisions*, as well as *engaging in mundane conversation*. For instance, to encourage Ana, Lily shared survivors' stories from a book she was reading as well as what she had heard about Farah Fawcett's (the actress) experience with remission.

All of these forms of behavior contributed to Ana's adjustment to cancer, but several were particularly helpful. Ana reportedly appreciated her mother's positive talk, which Lily enacted when her daughter expressed her anxiety about upcoming test results. Ana also felt that her mother's positive talk, which was in the form of reassurance, was instrumental in giving her faith and hope. She further indicated that she valued her mother's opinion and her maternal intuition. Ana was grateful when Lily validated her medical decisions and reassured her that the tests would turn out okay. These findings are consistent with those that emerged from daughters' interviews.

However, a new support behavior emerged: mundane talk was a salient presence. Although women were asked to include this aspect of their interactions in their diary entries, the striking presence of this type of talk is noteworthy. In her diary entries, Ana wrote about her mundane talk with her mother in positive ways. Lily referred to this talk as "our usual morning talk about what we were going to do the rest of the day." Often these interactions were pleasant, joyful, or fun. For instance, Ana liked talking to her mother about her children's activities. In turn, her mother liked hearing about her grandchildren. When Ana wrote about mundane conversations involving such topics, she usually also described having positive feelings (e.g., she wrote "nice conversation" or that they laughed together). Mundane talk did not emerge in the interview data prominently in this age group. In middle-adult- and later-life-diagnosed mothers' experiences (from interviews), participants reported that mundane conversation was a form of emotional support or a means of *staying normal.* During treatment, mundane talk may be particularly important as daughters adjust during treatment—a time at which cancer can literally be a pressing daily issue. Although Ana and Lily did not mention mundane talk with regard to normalcy, it is likely that this communication dynamic functioned in a similar manner by keeping things as they were in their bond even before Ana's diagnosis.

It is also important to consider that Ana's prognosis was more life threatening than most women's experiences. She was not only experiencing a severe stage (IV) and a recurrence, but she was also now in continuous treatment. Thus, the nature of Ana and Lily's coping experience may be particularly salient to those women facing a more life-threatening diagnosis or prognosis during young adulthood.

16

A PORTRAYAL OF COPING DURING MIDLIFE AS A DAUGHTER

Carrie is 44 years old. She describes herself as happily married with two children in their pre-teens. She works in the technology field full time, is an avid runner, and believes she has a supportive group of girlfriends. She was diagnosed with stage II breast cancer. She first underwent traditional chemotherapy treatment, then a mastectomy, and finally reconstruction. At the time of the study, she was undergoing another chemotherapy treatment with Herceptin, which is a form that has fewer side effects than conventional chemotherapy. As Carrie noted, "It doesn't make you sick or make you lose your hair, so people tend to think of it in different terms." She underwent the Herceptin treatment each week and had about 3 months left at the time that she journaled.

Her mother, Lorraine, is 64 and lives on the opposite side of the United States. She maintains an active lifestyle and lives with her ailing husband, Carrie's father. Lorraine is also the caregiver for Carrie's father, who suffers from Parkinson's disease. Carrie and Lorraine had lived a long distance apart for more than 10 years. They also had a family history of breast cancer. Although Lorraine has never been diagnosed, her mother is a survivor, and her sister and great-grandmother both died from the disease.

Carrie does not feel her relationship with her mother changed much following the diagnosis, whereas Lorraine feels they are closer. Carrie describes their relationship as a "typical" mother-daughter bond prior to the diagnosis. She did not portray her mother as a significant source of support before the diagnosis but did say she may vent to her from time to time. Her mother characterizes their bond as open. Carrie and Lorraine see each other a few times a year. However, they talk at least once a week via telephone. Carrie said that she initiates most calls because she is busier and would call when she had free time. Carrie had just been out to visit her mother a few weeks prior to the diary study.

During the two weeks of keeping a diary, Carrie and Lorraine communicated exclusively via telephone. Carrie called her mother twice a week. Their conversations lasted on average 24 minutes but ranged from 10 to 40 minutes. Carrie and Lorraine both wrote about three interactions occurring over the two weeks they journaled. Both women also indicated in the diary that they thought about cancer or cancer-related experiences that they did not share with each other for various reasons (Carrie had 6 entries and Lorraine 11). Carrie's diary entries were more in-depth and extensive in comparison to her mother's. Both participated in a diary interview about their journal entries.

OPENNESS DURING TREATMENT: DISCLOSED TOPICS AND REASONS FOR OPENNESS

Carrie and Lorraine mostly communicated about various topics unrelated to cancer: car trouble, Carrie's father's health, her mother's hobbies, Carrie's children, and other family members' activities. Carrie did discuss with her mother two cancer-related topics: *treatment side effects* and *diagnostic testing*. Her reasons for doing so were to *seek support* and *share good news*.

Carrie shared with her mother her experience with menopause-like symptoms. In her diary, she indicated that she talked about her concern that the symptoms might be a result of the traditional chemotherapy she received the previous year. She explained that her reason for disclosing this side effect was to attain her mother's support. She was also hoping her mother would share her experience with menopause. She thought that if her mother did this, she could develop greater insight into dealing with her own menopause. However, her mother did not respond as Carrie had hoped. Rather, she told her daughter that "for some people it's like that"

(Carrie's diary). Carrie did not ask her mother directly about her experiences with menopause and seemed to excuse her mother for not disclosing when she wrote, "If the doctor can't tell me if it's the cancer treatments or menopause, I don't know why I'd expect my mother to be able to!" Her mother did not write about this matter in her diary.

Carrie also shared with her mother experiences with medical testing. She talked to her mother about receiving genetic testing because of their family history of breast cancer. In addition, when she received a clear mammogram result, her first in 2 years, she immediately called her mother. She wrote that she wanted to "share the good news." When she finally did reach her mother, Carrie wrote that her mother "seemed relieved" when she told her the news. In the diary interview, Carrie explained that her mother's tone indicated to her that she was relieved and that her mother said something like, "That's good." Lorraine mentioned that conversation in her diary with more enthusiasm, writing, "We were both rejoicing together over the good mammogram results." Yet in her interview, Lorraine only described saying something like, "Oh great," to her daughter, with some enthusiasm, and then moving on to other topics.

In the diary interview, Carrie spoke in more detail about her feelings regarding her mother's response to her good news. Carrie admitted feeling a need to be allowed to be more open. She mentioned that her mother never brings up her cancer and does not talk about it much even when Carrie does. She noted that her mother "doesn't like to talk about it at length." Carrie admitted that she did not care if her mother brought the subject up but did not necessarily want her to. Still, at the same time, she did not understand her mother's response. She was not sure whether her mother did not like talking about the cancer or whether she was worried that talking about it upset her, but, for Carrie, it did not bother her to talk about it. In fact, Carrie felt that if she herself brought the subject up in conversation, it signaled to her mother that she did want to talk about it. Thus, by Carrie bringing it up herself, she did not necessarily want her mother to move on from the topic, as she felt her mother did. Carrie described her feelings about this, saying:

> She wants to end that part of the conversation probably quicker than I would like. . . . If I bring it up, there's usually something I really want to get off my chest—how I'm feeling about it. . . . When I start talking about it, I don't necessarily want to move on in the conversation—you know—[I want to] finish saying everything.

Carrie also referred to her mother's generally closed behavior with respect to health throughout her diary. She wrote that this behavior was how her family was. She had to "pull" information about health out of her mother and father. In fact, it was not until their conversation about genetic testing (described in the diary) that Carrie learned her great-grandmother had died of breast cancer.

Lorraine did not share this view. She felt they discussed Carrie's cancer openly, saying, "We cover it pretty thoroughly before we move on to something else. . . . That's a mutual [effort]." She also described wanting her daughter to talk about the subject. She mentioned not having open communication with her own mother or her sister after their diagnoses, and she even recalled her distress in having to "drag things out" of her sister. Lorraine felt her daughter knew to talk about her condition because she had complained to her about her sister not sharing with her in the past.

Although the diaries seemed to mirror the interview data, in that topics involve medical matters like *treatment side effects* and *diagnostic testing*, two new reasons for disclosure emerged from the diary (*seek support* and *share good news*). One of these reasons (*share good news*) had not yet emerged in any other age group's experiences in the interviews but had been a motive in the young-adult dyad diary. The first motive (*seek support*) did surface in young-adult daughters' accounts during interviews but not in those of middle-adult-diagnosed daughters'.

The diary findings highlight the complexity of open communication, particularly for midlife-diagnosed women with later-life moms. Although Carrie wanted to talk more openly about her cancer (and in more depth), she was understanding of her mother's closed and avoidant behavior and even described it as typical behavior across their relational history. Regardless of her understanding of her mom's closed behavior, Carrie voiced that she also wanted more openness from her mother. It is also important to note that her mother did not see herself as closed, nor did she feel they did not talk about her daughter's cancer in depth and, in fact, complained about the same closed behavior with her own mother and sister.

This finding may be more easily interpreted in consideration of generational differences in how individuals openly communicate. Each individual's characterization of openness, as well as need for disclosure, may differ. What Lorraine perceives as openness on her part might be quite open compared with what she experienced with her sister and her own mother given her identification of them as being closed off. Lorraine was satisfied with updates and described her daughter as being more open than her sister or mother. She also perceived that she was open with Carrie. She did not seem to understand that Carrie wanted and needed even more openness and depth in their discussions. Carrie is from a younger cohort who experienced a social history in which openness, particularly about health, was more readily accepted and encouraged. As such, Carrie may conceptualize openness differently than Lorraine and likewise have variant openness needs when coping.

A key aspect of open communication emerged (the daughter initiating cancer talk) that seemed to be a cue that the daughter wants to talk about it. To Carrie, such behavior should signal a desire and need for her mother to allow her to talk freely about her experience. It is also important to note that in the previous dyad's (Ana and Lily) experiences, like Lorraine, the mother (Lily) had mentioned *not* bringing up cancer because she was concerned it would upset her daughter. She allowed Ana to bring it up. Collectively these daughters' and mothers' stories demonstrate that midlife-diagnosed daughters need and want to talk openly, and mothers should be in tune to this particularly when the daughter initiates the topic. At the same time, daughters may need to bring it up more on their own given their mothers' hesitation in doing so as they also do not want their daughter to worry or stress unnecessarily.

AVOIDANCE DURING TREATMENT: AVOIDED TOPICS AND REASONS FOR AVOIDANCE

Carrie did not mention avoiding any cancer-related talk except for one issue: an *upcoming medical test* (a mammogram). She did not inform her mother that the test had been scheduled. Her reason was that she felt that her mother had already been through enough. Hence, she avoided this topic to *protect her mother*. She did not want to distress her. Carrie also wrote in her diary that she talked openly about her experiences with a woman she met at her weekly Herceptin treatment, sharing with her feelings regarding treatment. When asked during the diary interview why she openly communicated with this woman, Carrie stated that it was easier to talk to people who have been through cancer because they could understand her feelings better. This experience suggests that Carrie may have avoided disclosing to her mother, in part, because she *talked to others*. Both of these reasons (*protect mother* and *talk to others*) were in evidence in the interview data. However, in the interview data, "others" typically referred to loved ones, not less intimate acquaintances. This experience indicates that talking to other patients or survivors is something those with cancer want because of what they have in common, and this may be especially necessary while coping with treatment. As women are in treatment, they also have more interaction with other patients. This shared experience likely connects women, even strangers, on an immediately intimate level. Thus, the diary findings validate the interview results but also further illuminate the motivation behind daughters' avoidant behavior.

ENACTED EMOTIONAL SUPPORT DURING TREATMENT

Lorraine engaged in various types of emotional support during her daughter's treatment. She recalled *being humorous* and also *validating decisions* concerning genetic testing. Carrie described her mother *staying positive* to support her when she shared information about her medical tests. Such accounts were congruent with the interview findings within and outside this age group. *Validating decisions* did not emerge in this age group's interviews but frequently did with younger diagnosed daughters, both in the interview and diary-interview data.

Positive talk was the only behavior described in both adaptive and maladaptive terms. In the diary interview, Carrie indicated that her mother always responded to her in a positive manner. When asked whether this was always helpful, she said it was not. She recalled when she told her mother she had breast cancer. Her mother responded by saying that the cancer would not be a big deal, and it would probably involve nothing more than a lumpectomy. Carrie would have preferred a more emotional reaction in sync with her own. In a way, she seemed to want validation of her own emotions. Her mother's positive talk did not seem to make sense to Carrie in light of the seriousness of the diagnosis. Carrie said that she was feeling sad about the diagnosis, but her mother's response indicated to her that she was not feeling the same thing.

Although Carrie was reflecting on a past experience that did not occur during treatment, this account was consistent with the interview data. It also indicates an important detail in which mothers' positivity can be misinterpreted and even come across as hurtful. In this way, the findings extend the interview results and enhance our understanding of the context in which positively framed supportive communication can function maladaptively.

17

A PORTRAYAL OF COPING DURING MIDLIFE AS A MOTHER

Ellen is 50 years old with two teenage daughters. Her youngest is still in high school. Her oldest, Holly, was 18 and transitioning to college at the time of the study. Ellen feels her daughters are very different girls but is close to both of them. She describes herself as happily married. She runs a family business with her husband. Ellen was diagnosed with breast cancer (stage III) about 8 months prior to being interviewed. Since the diagnosis, her husband has worked later hours and, thus, is not home very often. Ellen had already undergone a mastectomy and was currently undergoing chemotherapy. She was nearing the end of treatment at the time of her diary entries.

Holly is a very active emerging-adult woman. At the time of the study, she was beginning her freshman year of college. She mentioned in the interview that she is very close to her mother and had a very hard time with the diagnosis in the beginning. After her mother's diagnosis, she and her mother both described her withdrawing from her mother. After Holly received therapy, both women thought Holly was doing better. Holly perceives that she both emotionally and instrumentally supports her mother in adjusting to breast cancer. She also shared that because her mother struggles with depression and runs a family business, Holly has always provided this type of social support to her mother. Her mother, however, perceived the nature of their supportive bond differently. Ellen does not perceive that Holly emotionally supported her in adjusting to cancer as much as her younger daughter. She found Holly to be more involved in instrumentally supporting her (e.g., around the house) and very helpful in doing so.

At the time of their diaries, Holly was moving to a dorm. Both Holly and Ellen seemed to be struggling with this new transition and their separation from each other. According to Ellen, Holly was very nervous about starting college. Yet from Holly's perspective, her mother was distressed about her leaving the house. From their diary entries, it appears that most of their interactions were face to face in their home. Only some communication took place by telephone. Holly initiated the communication more often. Their interactions lasted about 15 minutes on average when on the telephone and several hours when face to face. The communication time span ranged from a few minutes to half the day. Ellen wrote about nine interactions with her daughter. Holly wrote about 14. Both also made entries in which they reported thinking about cancer or having cancer-related experiences that they did not share with each other for various reasons (each had three such entries). At times, Holly's entries were slightly more detailed than her mother's. However, she rarely addressed emotion or how she was feeling whereas Ellen often did confront these experiences. Only Holly participated in a diary interview.

OPENNESS DURING TREATMENT: DISCLOSED TOPICS AND REASONS FOR OPENNESS

Many of Ellen and Holly's interactions took place at their home. Some communication also occurred at their family business, as Holly often helped Ellen with work. Like those in other dyads, most of their talk centered on topics unrelated to cancer. When Ellen mentioned cancer, it was in relation to *treatment side effects*. For instance, she shared with Holly that her neck was sore because of the chemotherapy. As in the interview data, openness about treatment side effects emerged. Although Ellen gave no reason for disclosing this matter, she did write about how much Holly's support meant to her.

Interactions centered mostly on Holly's life. A primary topic in both women's diaries was Holly's transition to college. The diary entries were recorded during the same weeks Holly was moving into a college dorm and beginning her freshman year. In the midst of cancer treatment, the pair was also experiencing a notable transition in the daughter's adulthood that was significant to them both.

AVOIDANCE DURING TREATMENT: AVOIDED TOPICS AND REASONS FOR AVOIDANCE

Holly and Ellen both actively avoided talking about cancer. As noted, they both had entries about their cancer-related thoughts that they consciously chose not to share with one another. Ellen wrote about her *emotional distress or negative affect*, which she hid from her daughter. For instance, she did not share with her daughter her emotional distress regarding a side effect from treatment ("chemo brain/fog"). In this instance, she and Holly were working together at the family business. Ellen was struggling with remembering things (because of the chemo fog) and was becoming distressed. Holly did not seem to understand what was wrong with her mother and was becoming impatient. Rather than explain to Holly what was wrong, Ellen tried to manage her distress on her own. In a similar diary entry, Ellen recalled being emotionally frustrated with still having to endure chemotherapy. She wrote, "Tomorrow I have my next to last chemo—I'm getting so tired of this! I didn't tell anyone because they need me to be strong. I cried in my room." Ellen also wrote about being concerned that she could not be more helpful to her daughter in her move to the dorm. She reported feeling fatigued and frustrated with her itchy wig in the summer heat. She also felt guilty because she perceived that her cancer was impeding on her daughter's life transition to college:

> I feel bad that she has to do so much on her own. My husband had to work late, and I can't lift much, so she had to load the car by herself. I felt like I let her down today because I couldn't be more helpful.

Ellen further noted becoming emotional during the move because she was so hot and frustrated with her physical limitations. However, she did not disclose to her daughter why she was upset. As a result, Holly may have misinterpreted her mother's behavior (as her mother felt she did at the family business). As Ellen recalled,

> We didn't talk much about my cancer, but during move-in, I got overheated, tired, and cranky. This wig is horribly hot, and it's 98 degrees outside! Holly got angry that I was cranky.

Like mothers in the interviews, Ellen avoided talking about the emotions she experienced that were related to cancer. She concealed these feelings because "they need me to be strong" and because she did not want Holly to worry. Hence, she avoided topics to *protect* Holly. Most of the time, this avoidance seemed to function maladaptively for both women. Ellen noted feeling emotionally overwhelmed and, at times, alone, whereas Holly became agitated because she misinterpreted her mother's behavior.

Interestingly, Holly often wrote about her cancer-related thoughts and her reasons for keeping them to herself. For example:

> I try not to mention much about my mom's illness because I don't want to make her think about it anymore than she already has to. I just try to live the life we had before she was diagnosed or as close to it as possible.

The pattern was evident in others' diaries. Like the mothers of diagnosed daughters, Holly did not bring up any cancer-related matters with her mother because she was concerned that talking about cancer would only upset her.

ENACTED EMOTIONAL SUPPORT DURING TREATMENT

The preceding quotation reflects how Holly emotionally supported her mother by *staying normal.* As was evident in the interview data, keeping things normal was important in mother-daughter dyads in this age group. In this diary case, much of their interactions focused on Holly's transition to college. The two went shopping for everything Holly needed and also had talks about Holly's fears. Ellen indicated how these interactions helped her adjust to the disease. She felt needed by Holly and, at the same time, *wanted* to mother her. This aspect of interaction emerged in the interview data as an important communicative pattern that mothers perceived as emotionally supportive. Mothers wanted to be kept in their daughters' lives, and they wanted their daughters to continue their lives as normal.

Consistent with this cohort of mothers' and daughters' interviews, Holly also attempted to be supportive by *staying positive* (e.g., reassurance), *showing affection* (e.g., hugs and massages), and *being there* (e.g., telling her mom she could count on her). Much of Holly's support was also instrumental. She drove her younger sister to her activities, did laundry, cooked dinner, and helped her mother manage the family business. Ellen wrote about the significance of this support as being emotionally helpful to her: "I told her how thankful I am to have her." Interestingly, the meaning of instrumental support to this midlife-diagnosed mother is also in line with diagnosed daughters in midlife. For women diagnosed in this period of life, instrumental help (from a mother or a daughter) may be particularly critical to their adjustment given that it enhances their ability to continue managing the "juggling act" of midlife.

18

A PORTRAYAL OF COPING DURING LATER LIFE AS A MOTHER

CASE STUDY 1

Sally is 57 years old, is happily married, and lives with her husband on the East Coast. Her two children are both grown adults. Her son recently married and lives several hours away. Her daughter, Marie, also lives at a distance and is in a long-term relationship. Sally currently works part time at a health clinic in finance but had previously run a family business passed down to her from her family. After her first diagnosis, she and her family decided to sell the business because it required too much time and energy to run. She had first been diagnosed with stage II breast cancer and underwent a mastectomy, chemotherapy, and radiation. Two years later, she learned of a recurrence (stage IV) and that the cancer had metastasized to her lungs. She was currently in continuous chemotherapy treatment, for which there was no end date.

Sally's daughter, Marie, is a young adult and 30 years old. She is finishing graduate school and in the process of moving to a state closer to her mother's home. Although she lives several hours away from her mother, Marie often visits on weekends.

The two women talk almost daily on the phone. When her mother was diagnosed the first time, Marie was in another country. She immediately returned, moved back in with her parents, and began caring for her mother. After the recurrence, Marie returned home more frequently and developed great concern for her mother's well-being. She worries about their not having much time left together. Sally describes Marie as an unconditional, primary form of support for her. Marie seems to be aware that she is very important to her mother. Although they had their ups and downs during Marie's teen and college years, both Marie and Sally feel that they have become more tolerant of each other and extremely close.

Marie was visiting her mother during the first week they kept the diary. Hence, most of their interactions were face to face. A limited number occurred via telephone. They each initiated calls to each other with the same frequencies. Interactions lasted about 10 minutes on average but ranged from a few minutes to several hours. Sally wrote about nine interactions with her daughter, whereas Marie wrote about five. This dyad did not include entries about everyday interactions or thoughts ostensibly as a result of each woman having personal time constraints (Marie was finishing up graduate school, and Sally was working). Both Sally and Marie's diary entries were comparable in terms of their depth and details. However, at times, Marie's were slightly more detailed. Both women participated in a diary interview.

OPENNESS DURING TREATMENT: DISCLOSED TOPICS AND REASONS FOR OPENNESS

Compared with what those in other diary case studies reported, Sally and Marie talked more about cancer. For the most part, Sally and Marie's interactions focused on how Sally was feeling. Sally openly talked about her *treatment side effects* with Marie. She shared her experiences with indigestion, edema, hair loss, and fatigue. She admitted that she disclosed these topics with her daughter because she was *seeking her support*, particularly her "positive thoughts."

Marie also recognized that her mother did not always feel well and that she was concerned for her well-being. She often asked her mother how she was feeling to make sure she was okay. One side effect that Marie wrote about was her concern about her mother's self-consciousness about her appearance because of the hair loss. She and her mother both indicated talking about a negative interaction Sally experienced with a family friend she saw in public. Sally told Marie how this friend stared at her strangely and ignored her, which she attributed to her hair loss. It made Sally uncomfortable, and she disclosed this to Marie to elicit her support. In her diary, Sally wrote about this experience in the following way:

> I feel like I stand out in a crowd. Although I like my short hair! . . . Marie said I should ask them why they are looking so strangely at me and say a "few choice" comments! Bottom line—I sometimes feel uncomfortable in a room of "healthy" people.

This experience mirrors the interview data. Mothers disclosed their treatment side effects to their daughters. However, this diary entry also reveals more emotional aspects of hair loss and the struggle later-life-diagnosed women endure with regard to body image or changes in their physical appearance. Sally's and Marie's diary entries support the idea that hair loss can be a very salient issue for women in later life. In addition, Sally's reason for openness (*seek support*) did not emerge in the interview data for this age group. However, it did in the other age groups, in both interview and diary data.

Marie frequently asked her mother how she was feeling. This inquisitive communicative behavior is likely linked to a reason mothers gave for openness in the interviews—that their *daughters want to know*. Diagnosed mothers' openness may be a reflection of how much daughters seek their mothers' disclosures. As Marie was in young adulthood (as opposed to emerging adulthood), her maturity may have been central to her more active communication in seeking her mother's disclosures.

AVOIDANCE DURING TREATMENT: AVOIDED TOPICS AND REASONS FOR AVOIDANCE

Sally seemed to be very open with Marie about cancer-related topics. However, she did admit to not disclosing about two matters with her daughter. First, she had received an upsetting test result suggesting that she might need dialysis. Sally did not share this information to protect Marie. She did not want to "alarm" her. Marie, she felt, was busy finishing her thesis, and such news would distract and upset her. Hence, she was *protecting* Marie by not disclosing, a reason that also emerged in the interview data for this age group. In addition, a newly identified pattern of avoidant topics (*unfavorable test results or bad news*) emerged. This category relates to avoiding sharing about *upcoming test results* (a topic that surfaced in the middle-adult daughter dyad diary case study). This topic could be considered a distressful topic, which did emerge as a topic of avoidance in the interview data. It is also noteworthy that Sally's cancer prognosis was much more life threatening, like Ana's situation (the diagnosed young-adult daughter). Sally was in a later stage, in continuous treatment, dealing with a reoccurrence, and cancer that had metastasized. Thus, the implications of such results are likely much more distressing.

ENACTED EMOTIONAL SUPPORT DURING TREATMENT

Sally and Marie wrote about various instances in which Marie enacted emotional support for her mother. Marie and Sally went shopping together, as well as to lunch, and spent time together at Sally's house. Hence, the support of *being there* was clearly present. Marie also provided support by *listening* to her mother when she shared her feelings about how she felt during the interaction with the friend who ignored her. Marie gave support by *offering suggestions* concerning how to deal with side effects as well as her mother's hair loss.

Additionally, *being humorous* occurred in relation to a side effect Sally was experiencing. When Marie and Sally were shopping, Marie joked with her mother about her runny nose, a side effect she sometimes experienced. Marie wrote in her diary about this:

> Her nose was very runny yesterday, which some days it is. We were shopping, and she was going in and out of the store, and she had to blow her nose a lot. We stopped for ice cream, and I said it was like having an old dog follow me around—as a joke. She laughed so hard! It is helpful I think to use humor to talk about her problems and symptoms, sometimes to make light of it. . . . Later in the day, she was telling the rest of the family what I said and how funny it was. I thought that was cute.

Marie also mentioned *staying positive* with her mother (in particular, reassuring her). In her diary interview, she admitted that she often did this when she did not know what else to do. This nevertheless seemed to be important to Sally's adjustment. Sally wrote in her diary about talking to Marie about side effects to get her "positive thoughts." Sally also noted Marie's showing affection when she was not feeling well and was experiencing problems with her blood pressure and edema in her feet. Sally indicated that made her feel loved: "She was very concerned, we hugged, and gave each other a kiss. . . . I am touched by how much she cares about my well-being. She goes out of her way to make sure I am comfortable."

The only instance in which Marie's support appeared not to be helpful was when she *offered a suggestion* to her mother about her hair. Both women wrote about this interaction. Sally wrote about Marie's asking her why she was wearing her wig. She recorded in her diary the following responses: "My head gets cold; I scare patients; my hair needs [to be] professionally cut." Sally also wrote about her feelings when Marie asked her this:

> Marie said I shouldn't care what people think. She agreed that my hair should be cut nicer. It needs to grow longer! She can't argue with me about the fact my head gets cold. I was a little upset because I hate people telling me how to wear my hair.

In her diary, Marie recorded that she asked her mother why she was wearing her wig because her real hair looked cute as it was. She was just curious. Her mother, she noted, explained that it scared people when she did not wear it and that her head was cold without it. Marie was aware that the interaction upset her mother and was distressed by that:

> She referred to a comment that I made about how her hair would look better if she styled it. I felt bad because I thought I had hurt her feelings. I said, "Oh well, you should wear whatever makes you comfortable."

These findings are consistent with interview results relating to supportive behavior (e.g., importance of humor, listening, being there, affection) and later-life-diagnosed mothers' emotionally charged struggles with physical appearance, most notably hair loss. At the same time, the entries also provide more information about how daughters' suggestions about their mothers' hair can upset the mothers, an issue that did emerge in this cohort's interviews. It seems that Marie meant no harm in what she said and that she was aware of her mother's self-consciousness concerning her hair. She also noted that she felt her mother's hair looked great and did not require a wig. Nevertheless, as in the interview data, these suggestions were not well received by the mother. Sally seemed to understand that Marie was encouraging her not to wear the wig, but she also did not want anyone—her daughter included—offering advice about her hair. This behavior may relate to women's sense of privacy, which seemed to be prominent in the interview data for this age group of women. It is, nonetheless, indicative of a problematic issue (hair loss) and supportive behavior (offering suggestions) that may not always be helpful to mothers in later life when managing their new physical appearance.

CASE STUDY 2

Olivia is 57 years old. She lives with her husband on the East Coast and was going to soon be returning to work full time in counseling. She found work stressful and was motivated to change that aspect of her career. Olivia has one child, a daughter (Cassie), to whom she is very close. Olivia was diagnosed with stage III breast cancer about 11 months prior to the interview and diary participation. She had undergone a lumpectomy, finished chemotherapy, and was currently in, but nearing the end of, radiation treatment.

Cassie is 21 and, therefore, an emerging adult. She lives several states away from her mother. She recently graduated from college and is working a summer job in the art field. She is also preparing to move back to her home state to begin a new job. After this move, she would only be several hours away from her mother. Because Cassie is Olivia's only child, Olivia felt that she had the opportunity to spend a lot of time with her while she was growing up. They both describe their relationship as having consistently been that way. They talk almost daily and are open with each other about their lives. However, Olivia admitted that she did not share intimate details about her life with Cassie relating to her father. Olivia believed that the three of them (herself, her husband, and Cassie) were very family-oriented and pointed out that they still did all of their vacations and other such activities as a family.

While keeping the diary, Olivia and her husband (Cassie's father) traveled to visit Cassie. Cassie also surprised Olivia with a visit to their cabin when Olivia and Cassie's father were vacationing there. Much of their interactions occurred face to face as these mini-vacations occurred during the first week of their diaries. Their remaining interactions took place via telephone. They were equal in respect to who initiated calls. Interactions via telephone lasted about 10 minutes on average but up to several hours when speaking face to face. Interactions ranged from several minutes to 5 hours. Olivia wrote about 18 interactions with her daughter, and Cassie journaled about 3. Both also had entries in which they described thoughts about cancer or had cancer-related experiences that they did not share with each other for various reasons (Olivia had 14 entries, and Cassie had 5). Olivia's diary entries included more detail than her daughter's. Both women participated in a diary interview.

OPENNESS DURING TREATMENT: DISCLOSED TOPICS AND REASONS FOR OPENNESS

Most of Olivia and Cassie's interactions centered on issues other than cancer. For instance, they talked a lot about Cassie's job, the upcoming move, and her friends. They also talked about Olivia's apprehension about going back to work. The cancer-related topics Olivia talked about with Cassie centered on either her experiences with *treatment procedures* or the *side effects* she encountered. For instance, Olivia talked openly with her daughter about the soreness she experienced near her arm and on her breast due to radiation. She explained that her reason for disclosure was because she *sought her daughter's support.*

> I told her about using a sock to help soften the seat belt on my shoulder since radiation had dried and burned the skin. I sought emotional support about what I was managing. I got it with an "Oh good" kind of response.

Later in the diary, Olivia described a similar interaction and wrote that she wanted Cassie's comfort. When asked in her interview whether this was a satisfying response, Olivia replied,

> Sometimes I wished she had focused to talk more. But yeah—it was just kind of I want to make this kind of a quick little report. . . . I think the total honest answer would be there probably have been times in the late part of radiation where it just all seemed to be very routine. . . . I wasn't wanting her to be thinking much about it as a mom, but probably as a, as a—she is such a supportive person it would have been nice to get more from her.

Olivia then explained that perhaps her daughter could "ask a question about it or keep the conversation going by repeating back [what I said]. . . . If I'm bringing it up, then maybe a follow-up question or more response." Interestingly, Cassie indicated in her diary numerous times that she thought about her mother's cancer. Sometimes she thought about how the cancer made her family closer or how proud she was of her mother. However, she never brought up or shared these thoughts with her mother.

Although these entries initially mirrored the interview data, they reveal important interactive information about the diagnosed woman's openness that emerged in two of the other diary case studies. When a woman brings up the subject of her disease (regardless of her age or whether she is the mother or daughter in the relationship), it means she is open to discussion and, more importantly, needs to talk about it. It seems imperative that their mother/daughter not only respond with emotional support but to help facilitate the disclosure (and show interest) by asking questions. Given that Cassie is still an emerging adult, her maturity level may have contributed to this dynamic as well.

AVOIDANCE DURING TREATMENT: AVOIDED TOPICS AND REASONS FOR AVOIDANCE

Although Olivia talked openly with her daughter regarding her cancer, she acknowledged also avoiding discussion about her disease in general. She stated that she avoided talking about her *health and treatment* (or *cancer in general*) when possible. She felt she only wanted to keep Cassie updated and tended to share more with her husband. Olivia's reason for avoiding cancer talk was to not burden Cassie. Hence, she was *protecting her daughter*. However, she also chose to *talk with others* (e.g., her husband). Olivia explained,

> I would say Cassie and I aren't as involved in cancer treatment talk and worries right now. I don't want this to be a big part of our talks together as other things are more important to me. From what she has said about the difference during surgery, chemo time, and radiation makes me believe she is less worried about me and how I'm doing. That's good.

Like other diagnosed mothers, Olivia is keenly aware of how her daughter is faring, and knowing that her daughter is okay makes her feel okay. Olivia prioritizes this in her discussions of what mother-daughter communication helps her cope. In this instance, the findings match well with the interview data on multiple levels (protecting daughter, talk with others) but also suggest that avoidance may function adaptively for mothers in midlife and, more specifically, for mothers with emerging-adult daughters, given that this age group of daughters tended to exhibit more distress because of their mothers' diagnosis. Olivia expressed that once her daughter seemed to be coping well, it was better not to discuss cancer all the time. This communication pattern, according to Olivia, enhances her own sense of well-being.

ENACTED EMOTIONAL SUPPORT DURING TREATMENT

Both Olivia and Cassie discussed various situations in which Cassie provided emotional support, including *offering suggestions, complimenting her mother's hair, listening, being humorous,* and *staying positive.* The first week of diary entries made reference to time together and enacted support from Cassie that seemed especially helpful for Olivia. This type of support was uplifting for Olivia, particularly when Cassie surprised her and joined her parents at their new cabin. Olivia also wrote about the joy she experienced in being with her daughter, as well as in having dinner with Cassie and her friends during a visit. Olivia often mentioned admiring her daughter's behavior and communication. She once wrote, "Pride and smiles all around," after a face-to-face visit. She seemed to be energized by spending time with her daughter as she wrote, "Being with my daughter and friend with such energy and enthusiasm is catching and energizes me." Consistent with the interview data, *spending time together* seemed particularly important to Olivia's adjustment. Olivia also wrote about receiving *affection* from her daughter quite often, and at one time she specifically indicated how meaningful this form of support was to her: "Her hug was so wonderful. They feel different to me now—last longer, more special. I remember my feelings about hugs changed with my diagnosis."

Another form of support about which Olivia and Cassie frequently wrote was Olivia's wanting to hear about Cassie's life and wanting to be involved in supporting her through her stresses of finding a new home and job. While this support may be construed as *staying normal*, it could also be a reversal of *being there* support, in that Olivia was *being there* to support her daughter. This support seemed to function adaptively for Olivia. As she recorded, "I want to help with [Cassie's move]. So it was kind of mutual support. I wanted to be with her as that is such a positive in my life." Later she wrote about another time Cassie shared her personal life: "I loved hearing about her day!" Like diagnosed mothers' experiences depicted in the interview data, engaging in her role as a mother appears to be critical to Olivia's disease coping and well-being.

These findings reinforce those in the interview showing more depth in how support in the forms mentioned proved to be helpful in mothers' adjustment. They also reveal that the diagnosed women can be actively involved in eliciting emotional support. For instance, Olivia actively sought to be involved in her daughter's life because being involved helped her feel needed. Still, in line with the interview data, mothers with emerging-adult daughters are particularly concerned for their daughter's well-being, and knowing they are coping okay allows the mother to enhance her own well-being as well.

CONCLUDING THOUGHTS AND IMPLICATIONS OF TRIANGULATING DATA

By collecting women's mother-daughter coping stories through individual in-depth interviews, longitudinal daily diaries, and interviews about their diaries, a more intricate portrait emerges of how mother-daughter communication is central to women's wellness after a breast cancer diagnosis. Using three distinct qualitative methods to capture mothers' and daughters' lived experiences allowed for a deeper understanding of mother/daughter coping preferences and needs at various points in the life span, the nature of how they share the disease experience in an effort to cope together and at times separately, and how their communicative behaviors can both enhance and inhibit their ability to adjust in a healthy manner. An over-arching theme inherent in these women's lives was that it didn't matter who was diagnosed in the relationship—mothers and daughters are concerned for each other and prioritize the other's well-being in making sense of their own needs and wellness.

The diary and diary-interview findings serve as an excellent tool in qualitative research in which to validate findings sought via other methods and to extend them by situating the investigation of behavior within one realm of the experience. In this case, the focus of mother-daughter communication was during the treatment phase of the cancer trajectory, which may prove to be the most difficult time mothers and daughters must learn to cope with. While the diary findings mirrored and, thus, matched interview findings in each age group, analyses also expanded knowledge of mother-daughter communication in a more meaningful way.

For instance, by journaling, mothers and daughters could illustrate more of the interactive nature of their experiences and more in-the-moment behavior. As such, this method also captured the interactive nature of the three communicative behaviors analyzed separately in the interviews. The journals captured how interconnected openness and emotional support are in mothers' and daughters' communicative experiences. One particular noteworthy issue was that the mothers and daughters of diagnosed women tended *not* to bring up the cancer. Openness was left up to the diagnosed woman. Yet when diagnosed women did openly discuss cancer-related issues, their mothers and daughters did not always respond in ways that cultivated an open interaction (e.g., didn't respond much, show interest, or ask questions). Diagnosed women admitted wanting their mothers/daughters to allow them to talk openly as they were also seeking some form of emotional support. Some also felt that by not bringing it up, they buffered their loved one from stress, but in other instances, women felt that not bringing it up ignored the issue. The dialectic of openness and closedness was complicated for daughters and mothers and clearly a predecessor to attaining support needed to cope with stressors. This may be particularly important when women are still in cancer treatment. It may also be especially salient for women dealing with more life-threatening cancer experiences. All but one of these women were diagnosed with late stages of cancer (III or IV), two were in continuous treatment due to recurrences or metastases, and two were considered elevated or high risk for the disease (given their family history of breast cancer or a positive test result for a BRCA gene mutation).

Additionally, some mother-daughter communication not identified during interviews seems particularly relevant when experiencing treatment. In particular, the presence of mundane talk was important. Women tended to talk most about other aspects of their lives (e.g., children, grandchildren, moving to college, etc.). The diaries and diary interviews demonstrate that talk about women's daily lives that is not related to cancer can be a significant aspect of their coping adjustment during treatment, likely providing a sense of normalcy or balance for their relationships and their individual lives. Furthermore, for diagnosed mothers, it can be a means of allowing them to continue in their role as mother to their daughter, which clearly was important to their healthy disease coping and adjustment. Everyday chatter provides the women a sense of connection to each other in other aspects of their lives. It allows a mother to be a mother to her daughter and for a daughter to be mothered. Ultimately, this communicative act conveys that "life still goes on." For diagnosed mothers, this seems particularly important as it helps them know their daughters are okay (making them feel better) and also allows mothers to feel needed by their daughters.

Finally, the diary case studies showed the influence of human development on mother-daughter communication. For instance, the findings depict the complexity of open communication and avoidance, particularly for diagnosed women with later-life mothers or emerging-adult daughters. For these daughters, emerging adulthood appears to be an important period in which much maturity in communication competence and understanding is attained. This is certainly in line with Arnett's (2000) work that distinguishes emerging adulthood (the 20s) from young adulthood (the 30s). Although the daughters' age difference was only about a decade, much growth occurs during a woman's 20s. Daughters in their 30s typically exhibited a level of maturity in attending to or being able to perceive their mother's needs a bit more than the emerging-adult daughters. As such, it seems important for mothers to consider their daughter's developmental maturity when interpreting their behavior.

Additionally, for women diagnosed in midlife, it was especially critical to them that their mothers be open to talking about breast cancer. Given that their mothers are older and of a generational history in which openness, and especially talk about cancer, was not encouraged, this may not come so easily. In fact, their aging mothers may think they are being open, as was evidenced in the midlife-diagnosed daughter-mother case study. More understanding for both mother and daughter is needed on each woman's unique, generationally influenced open communication preferences. Likewise, it may be difficult for daughters of diagnosed women in later life to understand that their mothers do not want to discuss cancer as openly as they do, which again may be tied to their inclinations for being less open or, as many framed it, a need for more privacy.

Collectively, the triangulation of findings helps to further demonstrate the important role of context in mother-daughter communication when coping with breast cancer. As Goldsmith (2004) asserted, the context of communication matters, particularly if we are to understand how our family behavior can function both adaptively and maladaptively in our ability to manage cancer-related stress, renegotiate identity and relationships, and maintain wellness. A woman's age or human development matters, as do her relational role of mother or daughter and the topic of conversation or course of disease. Without context, it is not possible to fully capture necessary conditions for communication to function in healthy ways. These women's beautiful stories are a critical component to understanding how mothers and daughters can join together to cope resiliently. And the research design used, triangulating stories from multiple methods, more comprehensively illustrates how mothers and daughters can emerge from breast cancer strengthened, both individually and relationally.

Table 18.1 Diary Case Study Analyses: Triangulating Findings

To effectively cope in this type of mother-daughter bond during treatment	*diagnosed women share these topics*	*for these reasons,*	*and avoid these topics*	*for these reasons,*	*and receive this support when coping together.*
young-adulthood diagnosed daughter-mother bond	treatment side effects medical decisions diagnostic testing & results**	seek support share good news* protect mothers	distressful topics	protect self	being humorous staying positive validating decisions mundane talk*
middle-adulthood diagnosed daughter-mother bond	treatment side effects diagnostic testing & results	seek support** share good news*	upcoming tests*	protect mother talk to others	being humorous staying positive validating decisions**
middle-adulthood diagnosed mother-daughter bond	treatment side effects	-----	negative affect	protect daughter	showing affection staying normal staying positive being there*
later-adulthood diagnosed mother-daughter bond	treatment side effects & procedures	seek support*	unfavorable test results/bad news* cancer in general*	protect daughter talk to others	listening showing affection being humorous being there/staying normal staying positive offering suggestions spending time together giving compliments

*Denotes emergent patterns in diary analyses that were not recurrent in interview data.
**Denotes emergent patterns new to that age group but emergent in another age group's interview data.

Part VIII

ENHANCING MOTHERS' AND DAUGHTERS' "PSYCHOSOCIAL MAP" OF BREAST CANCER

19

EXTENSIONS AND PRACTICAL IMPLICATIONS OF THE FOUNDATIONAL STUDY

I could always count on her.
Diagnosed Daughter

You've got me, and I've got you.
Mother to Her Diagnosed Daughter

What is clear from these narratives is that breast cancer impacts not only the diagnosed woman but her mother and daughter. As they navigate these often choppy waters, they unite together and work to find balance, peace, and happiness, all while striving to be there for one another. These women's shared stories help illustrate that the path is not altogether easy, but that the mother-daughter connection is incredibly resilient and, ultimately, a force in women's wellness and survival.

Since the foundational study, I have embarked on numerous extensions of this research, both with secondary analyses of the data as well as extensions of the findings through new ongoing studies, some of which involve collaborations with Mayo Clinic (Arizona) and Memorial Sloan-Kettering Cancer Center (New York). With this collective body of research in mind, I offer some final thoughts on the nature of breast cancer as a turning point in the mother-daughter bond. I also re-address some prominent issues that mothers and daughters might encounter after a diagnosis, with associated practical guidance for clinicians and families, and end with some factors to consider in future research.

A TIME OF RELATIONAL CHANGE: POINTS OF NEGOTIATION

As discussed in the first two chapters, breast cancer is a turning point for mothers and daughters and can become a critical juncture in their relational history. Fundamentally, this transition is a point of negotiation for mothers and daughters and, therefore, a chance to improve how they relate to one another. Although their joint coping journey will not be without some bumps along the road, how mothers and daughters communicate is central to their ability to understand where each woman is coming from with regard to her individual concerns and coping preferences in managing breast cancer-related stress.

On a most basic level, it seems particularly important that mothers and daughters make an effort to "be there" for each other and, at the same time, be aware of and manage their own individual needs. For many diagnosed women, simple changes in their mother-daughter communication dynamics were a fundamental sign that the other woman cared. For instance, talking more (whether it be by phone, email, text, Skype, or in person) and making more of an effort to spend time together (on a day-to-day basis or with more long-distance trips/visits) means a lot to diagnosed women and, in turn, helps their mothers and daughters cope by allowing them to "be there" and see that their loved one is okay (Fisher & Nussbaum, 2012). For some women, this may be new territory—spending more time together and talking more—and for others it may already be a prominent feature of how they relate to one another. Regardless, when mothers and daughters sense the other is making an *effort*, they feel loved and supported.

When these basic changes in relational communication occur, women at times also encounter more open dialogue, whether it be about cancer or aspects of their personal lives (Fisher & Nussbaum, 2012). Women sometimes feel a natural transition to let each other "in" a bit more, whereas others may struggle to redefine their relational boundaries. With these changes comes increased intimacy and, for some mothers and daughters, a relational redefinition. At times diagnosed women described this as seeing "another side" of their mother or daughter, one they had not yet experienced. Many women believed these communicative changes allowed them to understand one another more so, leading them to become more tolerant and accepting of their mother or daughter as well as less controlling or manipulative.

Still, as we learned from these mother-daughter stories, enacting helpful emotional support is not easy nor is it always comfortable to open up, let alone really listen to and hear the other person's disclosure. This may be markedly so for mothers and daughters who do not have a prior history of encouraging openness in their bond or being mutually supportive. As discussed in Chapter 8, the Revised Family Communication Patterns instrument used in this foundational study could prove to be a useful tool for clinicians working with families' psychosocial coping needs. Given the importance of openness and support, this tool can help practitioners identify those individuals who may need more guidance and insight about opening up with their loved ones after a diagnosis or those individuals who may need access to other supportive outlets.

In essence, while breast cancer can be a profound turning point of growth uniting mothers and daughters, the path is complicated. Because these women generously shared some of their most beautiful, frustrating, upsetting, and heart-warming experiences with their own mothers and daughters, we have a better sense of how they can engage in healthier openness and emotional support communication. Thus, we have a better sense of the communicative behaviors needed for mothers and daughters to cope resiliently.

It may be particularly important for families to consider some of the issues highlighted in the rest of this chapter. Intertwining these issues is the prominent role our developmental place in life plays in our family health experiences. It seems crucial that mothers and daughters (and families as a whole) enhance their awareness of how age or human development is an important factor in facilitating healthy communication.

To Be or Not to Be Open . . .

Being open with one another after a cancer diagnosis (whether it be about cancer or not) may not only enhance mothers' and daughters' relational health but buffer diagnosed women from cancer-related physical ailments such as pain or fatigue (Fisher et al., 2013; Fisher, Fowler, & Wolf, in process). Yet using a communication lens, one can appreciate that just being open is not so simple and not always the answer. Diagnosed women often do not disclose because they want to protect their mother or daughter or buffer her from what they perceive as unnecessary distress. A strong desire to protect one another is clearly a resilient feature of the mother-daughter bond. This motivation to disclose or not makes sense and likely functions adaptively for mothers and daughters in many cases. However, what women also want to keep in mind is that by not disclosing, their mothers and daughters sometimes feel more uncertain, scared, or "kept in the dark." Essentially *not knowing*, or not disclosing, might contribute to women, particularly emerging-adult daughters, viewing cancer and their loved one's health as much more frightening and confusing. As a result, the motivation to not disclose to protect one's mother or daughter can backfire.

It is also important to consider that women enter the world of illness with their own pre-existing personalities, conditions, and preferences in communicating. Diagnosed women sometimes expressed that they knew what type of information their mother/daughter could handle based on personality or past history with medically related issues. At times women shared that they monitored what they disclosed because they were aware of a mother/daughter's previous struggles with depression or anxiety disorders. In such cases, the motivation to protect may be particularly important given that women, at times, experience distress as a result of the diagnosed woman's disclosures.

Moreover, diagnosed women can encounter the same distress after disclosing. It is less common for their mother/daughter to bring up any cancer-related topic, often for fear that it may upset the diagnosed woman. Still some diagnosed women experienced less satisfying responses from their mother or daughter when sharing fears or concerns, leading them to feel further silenced or not cared for (e.g., the mother/daughter changed the subject or appeared uninterested). It is important that their mother/daughter recognize certain behavioral cues (e.g., the diagnosed women initiates the conversation about cancer) as a signal that their loved one wants or needs to talk. In light of these experiences, it is also important that diagnosed women access other forms of familial or intimate bond support (e.g., a spouse, sibling, or close friend) but also to consider less familiar relationships. For instance, some diagnosed women felt that, at times, they needed the support of an "outsider" to their family but an "insider" to their health experience—in other words, a woman who had been through it before (i.e., a survivor or patient).

In the end, the dilemma to disclose or talk openly is difficult and depends on a number of individual and contextual factors. It is important to consider the uniqueness of each individual woman and balance what is shared and what is kept private. To ensure each woman's needs and preferences are contemplated and understood, mothers and daughters should consider engaging in frank conversations about how much they want to hear and what they do not feel comfortable talking about or sharing and realize that these preferences may change across the course of the disease.

Some notable developmental differences are also important to keep in mind. In considering individual differences, daughters with later-life-diagnosed mothers may want to be understanding of their need for privacy. Perceptions about openness vary across generational cohorts. Consequently, daughters and mothers may differ in their openness preferences. Older women are less likely to be expressive, and this may be especially true when the topic is cancer, given they experienced a social history when the disease was highly stigmatized and families were silenced. Dr. Sandra Petronio's evidence-based Communication Privacy Management (CPM) theory may also be particularly insightful (see Petronio, 2013, for a recent update on the theory; Caughlin & Petronio, 2004). Developed over more than 30 years of research, Petronio's theory helps us understand how patients "own" their illness information. It is *their* choice what to disclose and what to keep private. Moreover, according to CPM theory, later adult women may perceive their diagnosis and treatment as a "conventional secret," meaning they perceive it as inappropriate to talk about openly but not necessarily wrong to discuss. At the same time, however, the openness/privacy dialectic is a timeless feature of the mother-daughter relational history. It is an unending issue of boundaries, control, and intimacy they struggle to balance across the entire life span. Therefore, aging mothers may just want to keep some aspects of their lives separate from their daughters.

All women describe a tension between wanting to share their experiences and needing to protect their mother/daughter. A relational dialectics theoretical perspective (RDT) can, therefore, be insightful in future research (see Fisher, 2011, for a review of dialectical tensions experienced when coping as well as Dr. Leslie Baxter's, 2011, renowned work on RDT). Still this tension may be an exceptionally challenging issue for women diagnosed in midlife who are literally stuck in the middle. They may have the tension on both ends (as a mother and a daughter). They may want and need that support of their mother/daughter but also do not want to "lay that much on." Some midlife daughters expressed frustration with their aging mothers not allowing them to talk as much as they wanted, and midlife mothers sometimes felt their young daughters were being too self-focused when they did not want to hear about their mothers' cancer experiences. At the same time, midlife-diagnosed women struggle with how much to actually share with their mother/daughter. They are concerned it could exasperate aging mothers' prior issues with anxiety or sadness or that their young daughters could develop such distress. This tension between open and closed communication may lead to midlife-diagnosed women's own needs becoming silenced. As Fingerman, Nussbaum, and Birditt (2004) note about women in this age period, "[They] may be forced to focus so much on other people. . . . Their ability to communicate their own needs may become stifled" (p. 145). In the face of breast cancer, it is especially urgent that mothers and daughters are aware of this tension so that the midlife-diagnosed woman's individual needs are not sacrificed.

Understandably, midlife-diagnosed women with emerging-adult daughters may sacrifice their own needs in light of their daughters becoming quite distressed, as was evident with many of the mothers and daughters in this research. Daughters' refusal to communicate is not only a marker of distress and poor adjustment but inhibits mothers' ability to cope effectively (Fisher, 2010). A daughter's extreme withdrawal and avoidance can compete with her mother's desire to talk in an effort to communally cope. This pattern emerged during coping but also during discussions about daughters' disease prevention—an issue mothers often felt a burning need to discuss. Given the maladaptive nature of this coping response for daughters and mothers' extreme concern for their daughter's well-being, I have engaged in several lines of research to better understand how to enhance their joint coping.

Follow-up studies conducted in collaboration with Mayo Clinic (see Fisher, Pipe, Wolf, & Piemonte, 2012, in process; Fisher, Pipe, Wolf, Piemonte, & Canzona, 2012, in process) reveal that facilitating a healthier mother-emerging adult daughter communication environment is critical to *both* women's adjustment. To manage this tug-of-war experience, both women must employ new communication strategies. We have found that daughters feel more comfortable talking to their mothers when they reframed the purpose or value of the conversation. For instance, it was important that daughters consider how they could use the opportunity to provide support to their mothers for the first time in their bond. Many felt a sense of fulfillment in being able to "be there" for their mothers. Daughters also looked more positively at mother-daughter interactions when they realized it was an opportunity to address their own concerns. They could gain information to reduce their own uncertainty (making it less scary) and better understand their mother's needs. At the same time, it is critical that mothers be the ones to initiate the conversation but also keep it brief, use a calm tone and keep the conversation light (not too serious), frame talks with a positive outlook, use humor when necessary to lighten the mood, and ensure they talk about life other than cancer (do not make it about cancer all the time). When talking about the daughters' health-promotion behavior or minimizing future disease risk, mothers and daughters found it helpful if the conversation was more casual than serious in nature. Relatedly, daughters also did not want their mothers mentioning their feelings of guilt for having "passed on" the risk to their daughters. Timing was also important. Moms needed to initiate the conversation (but not talk about it all the time) and be willing to answer questions. Some moms felt that an opportune time was an indirect conversation in response to a commercial or television program—in other words, using someone else's experience to get the conversation going.

Ultimately, these women's experiences help show that communication is enacted and embedded within a context and that communication is inherently a developmental phenomenon. While negotiating openness after a diagnosis is a journey for mothers and daughters, so too are their attempts to be supportive.

To Be or Not to Be Supportive . . .

As was evidenced in these women's recollections, some support communication seems to function in a helpful manner consistently regardless of the mothers' and daughter' ages. Being there to listen (without response or empathetically), using humor, and showing affection both verbally (saying "I love you") and nonverbally (giving a hug) all seem to be key types of support critical to facilitating healthy coping and resilience (Fisher, 2010). These forms of emotional support were also predominantly important for coping with emotionally charged changes (e.g., managing body image, hair loss, and uncertainty). Given that women framed these behaviors as always supportive regardless of age, mothers and daughters may be especially competent in this type of communication or, in line with socioemotional selectivity theory, in fulfilling each other's emotionally focused needs. Barbee and colleagues' (1998) work on solace support in the context of coping with AIDS or HIV has shown that the most helpful support is often "solace behavior" (Barbee et al., 1998). Solace behavior centers on emotional needs and aims to emit positive emotional responses while expressing relational intimacy. Giving affection, doing things to enhance their spirits (e.g., humor), and listening are all behaviors that allow a woman space to express her feelings and to connect with her mother or daughter (see also Dr. Kory Floyd's work on the health benefits of expressive affection: www.koryfloyd.com).

Still, the nature of how mothers and daughters attempt to "be there" for one another is not without tensions, and this can be explained, in part, with an awareness of diversity in preferences due to one's place in the life course (see Fisher, 2010). For mothers with daughters diagnosed in young adulthood, it may be chiefly imperative to be conscious of a tension of connection and autonomy. These daughters need their mothers and, oftentimes, want them there with them. However, daughters also need to be the person setting the tone for how their mother will "be there" for them. The young-adult-diagnosed woman must have the "control" in the negotiation of how her mother shares the disease experience with her. Young-adult daughters' sense of independence is acutely vital for them given their place in the life cycle, and this can be challenging for mothers who also need to be there and "mother" their daughters for their own personal healthy coping.

While most forms of emotional support may function in both helpful and unhelpful ways, positivity may be especially complicated. For many mothers and daughters, it is a philosophy of life or a way of living ingrained in their family culture. Yet it proved to not always be helpful in women's disease adjustment. This may be further complicated given the prominence of and bias toward positivity in modern-day society. Being and thinking positively has become a prevalent social moral norm and is often perceived as fundamental to surviving cancer in popular culture (Wilkinson & Kitzinger, 2000). As a result, cancer patients encounter "moral and psychological pressure to 'think positively' about their disease" (de Raeve, 1997, p. 249). In fact, some patients seek help from psychologists and other mental health professionals fearing they are not positive enough (Gray & Doan, 1990).

In consideration of these women's stories and previous research on breast cancer patients' coping, what may be most critical is that positive support not *restrict* communication or be *unrealistic* (Chalmers, Thomson, & Degner, 1996). Secondary analyses of the data support this idea (see Fisher, Miller-Day, & Nussbaum, 2013). Positive emotional support is helpful when it provides a sense of hope or faith, reframes a person's perspective, calms fears, and offers reassurance. Moreover, women must also be certain that, by communicating positively to their mother or daughter, they are not also silencing her. Positivity is often juxtaposed with negativity. As a result, one may feel the need to replace negative talk with positive talk. However, mothers and daughters need the opportunity to vent and release concerns. It is crucial that positive communication not inhibit this. Thus, some "negative talk," as mothers and daughters called it, can be healthy. It can be helpful for diagnosed women to talk about fears and concerns or to release their sadness and anger. Releasing such emotions is beneficial in coping with an illness. It may be helpful to recall that disclosing in and of itself is healthy. Even negative talk can be an opportunity for women to disclose and release difficult feelings. In turn, when a diagnosed woman releases her fears and concerns, it can be an opportunity for her mother/daughter to empathize with her, show concern, and validate her feelings. Positivity may then follow it, as a means of being lifted back up.

A Diagnosed Woman's Role as Mother or Daughter

Regardless of whether the diagnosed woman was the mother or daughter in this maternal bond, they shared many of the same experiences in their cancer-related concerns, communication dynamics, and shared experiences of coping. Still some issues stand out specific to the diagnosed woman's relational role.

For diagnosed daughters coping with their mothers, a sense of independence or autonomy was an important feature of healthy coping. Namely, daughters needed to be in control of how their mothers coped with them. They also needed to feel that their mothers cared—they still needed a mother, essentially. At times, this was achieved from reassurances or validation support (e.g., with medical decisions or feelings and concerns), and in others it was from having open dialogue or consistency in being there. For daughters, an uncertain future (whether it be with regard to one's mortality, recurrence, or future life opportunities) was an especially challenging issue they needed support with. Relatedly, it seemed important for daughters to have their mother's intuitive faith that their daughter was going to be okay (and to hear their mothers voice this).

For diagnosed mothers coping with their daughters, a most central feature to their healthy coping was that the mother sensed that the daughter was making an effort to be there or cope together. They wanted time together—shared moments—that characterized their relational connection separate from cancer. While mothers struggle a bit more with the changes they endured to their physical appearance, daughters' support in this realm could be key to their management of difficult emotions. However, it was critical that daughters allow mothers the control in their disclosures and choices, recognizing their mothers' need for privacy. At the same time, mothers seem to cope better when family life continues "normally." They need to continue being their daughter's mother, and daughters too need their mothers' nurturance in their life separate from cancer.

There are many issues that still need to be intricately examined to continue to foster healthy mother-daughter breast cancer coping. However, several matters have stood out to me and have been consistently addressed in my own conversations with families, clinicians, and other behavioral scientists or social science scholars. I close with a few comments about these concerns with regard to future research.

MOVING FORWARD

In moving research forward and continuing to enhance mothers' and daughters' psychosocial map of coping, researchers, clinicians, and interventionists must try to enhance care with evidence-based practice. To contribute to research that can be used in this way, three notable issues warrant further attention.

First, a family's medical history and genetic make-up impact the nature of mothers' and daughters' breast cancer experiences (see also Gaff & Bylund, 2010). When women have a family history of the disease, they typically have a more heightened concern of disease risk. If they have lost family members to the disease (or know of familial losses), then they may have more dire expectations after receiving a diagnosis or hearing about their mother's/daughter's prognosis. This can also be greatly exasperated when they have determined a genetic association by testing positive for a BRCA gene mutation. Ultimately, these mothers' and daughters' familial culture is unique and warrants special consideration in how their mother-daughter needs might be different. In my collaborative research with Memorial

Sloan-Kettering Cancer Center, we have looked at the role of uncertainty in high or elevated risk mothers' concern for their daughters. They are uncertain as to how to talk about many things (e.g., screening) as well as their own and their daughter's risk (Bylund et al., 2012). At the same time, they need help communicating with their daughters and want them included in medical appointments (Fisher et al., 2014), suggesting a need for more research on provider-patient-family communication with families that are considered at high or elevated risk.

Second, culture is too often ignored in both health research and family studies. Relational research has shown that mothers and daughters communicate differently depending on cultural expectations and norms (Rastogi & Wampler, 1999). Moreover, culture plays a role in women's cancer experience, health promotion behavior, and reception of messages from their family and outside sources (see the work of Kreuter et al., 2000, 2007, 2008). Moreover, they may have different expectations and norms with regard to communicating health-related information. It is important to ascertain how mothers' and daughters' coping experiences, preferences, and needs may be similar but also unique across various cultures, especially in designing health messages for interventions that will be efficacious in educating families and teaching healthy behavior.

Finally, how we define "family" in our clinical practice and research is important. As Galvin, Bylund, and Brommel (2004) assert, "There are many ways to be a family." A notable limitation with the socioemotional selectivity research is that family is conceptualized in structural, legal, or biological terms (aunt, grandson, sibling) without specific attention to other ties one may perceive as family, although not in a legal or biological sense. Only a handful of women in this study were of nonbiological ties. Yet their inclusion demonstrates that the way we define "family" needs to be done more holistically. It may also be important to consider how various maternal bonds (e.g., adopted dyads, custodial grandmother-granddaughter, surrogate mother such as a close friend or an aunt, stepmother-daughter or blended families, daughters of same-sex or gay parents) may function uniquely in women's coping.

While these are only a few issues warranting careful consideration in future lines of research, it is also vital that scholars embark on research that is suited for translational purposes. As was noted early in this book, my research on mother-daughter communication and breast cancer coping has been done with the intention of producing knowledge useful for enhancing clinical practice and intervention-making. In the final chapter of this book, I encourage the translation of this research into clinical practice, training, and psychosocially focused interventions and resources with the aim of enhancing mother-daughter communication in family life, the quality of their oncology care, and patient health outcomes.

20

TRANSLATING RESEARCH TO PRACTICE

It may take as long as one or two decades for original research to be put into routine clinical practice. Thus, the translation of research findings into sustainable improvements in clinical practice and patient outcomes remains a substantial obstacle to improving the quality of health care.
U.S. Dept. of Health & Human Services (see AHRQ, 2001)

The National Institutes of Health (NIH) has identified "translational research" as a major priority. An NIH special interest group, Translational Research Interest Group (TRIG), bridges research and practice to improve patient care, and, for nearly 30 years, NIH's National Cancer Institute's (NCI's) Community Clinical Oncology Program has helped facilitate collaborative research between community oncologists and scientists to ensure that research is translated into evidence-based practice. For almost 10 years, funding for translational research and training has been covered by the NIH Common Fund, which was enacted into law by Congress through the 2006 NIH Reform Act. These federal initiatives collectively advocate for scientists to be concerned with not just generating knowledge about illness, health care, and quality of life, but to care about how that information is then used to improve the health of society. As renowned health communication researcher and founding chief of the Health Communication and Informatics Research Branch at the NCI, Dr. Gary Kreps, asserted, "There appears to be greater focus by many scholars on the process of conducting and reporting health communication research than on actually applying the results of relevant health communication research to enhance health-promoting practices and policies" (2012, p. 6). This task is, perhaps, the most critical to tackle—how knowledge generated by research can be disseminated and implemented to improve family life and health outcomes.

To translate research to clinical practice or behaviorally focused interventions, three stages of translation (awareness, acceptance, and adoption) are critical (Green & Siefert, 2005). In this vein, and after multiple requests and recommendations from the mothers and daughters participating in my studies, I sought to not only publish this book but to establish a research program website (www.motherdaughterbreastcancer.com) designed to connect the scholarship with clinicians, scientists, and community support resources, as well as families facing breast cancer. This book of mother-daughter coping stories is also a translational effort and may serve to disseminate knowledge and, therefore, heighten *awareness* of how our familial communicative behavior is central to wellness in the midst of breast cancer. Yet we must ensure *acceptance* of this knowledge (by both clinicians and families) and help mothers and daughters *adopt* healthy coping interactions. This book may serve as a guide for mothers and daughters in *adopting* healthier communication when coping with breast cancer. However, to ensure the research is actually translated in this manner, the development of psychosocial interventions and resources are direly need. This is particularly important in the clinical setting in which oncology care is provided.

There are, no doubt, many avenues one could take in translating this research to practice. However, given my storied approach to research, it seems best to apply this mother-daughter tapestry of lived experiences to interventions and education that draw on narratives to enact behavior change and facilitate medical training.

THE HEALING POWER OF STORY

Breast cancer storytelling is a relatively common entity in today's world and can take many forms. Each year we see new survivors' first-hand accounts depicted in popular press books as well as intense photography exhibits that selflessly invite us into women's cancer journeys. Society also encounters a multitude of theatrically driven illness stories, ranging from mainstream movies and portrayals in primetime televisions series (e.g., NBC's *Parenthood*) to documentaries such as Joanna Rudnick's *In the*

Family, in which she tells her own story of living with the BRCA1 gene mutation and the difficult decisions she faced to minimize her risk as a young adult.

Storytelling is also used to connect science with the real world. Social scientists have used the "power of the arts as an exceptional learning tool for extending empirical research" (Beach et al., 2013, p. 1; see also Ellingson's, 2009, crystallization methodology on merging social science analyses with creative representations). Narratively driven educational programs and interventions have been developed to improve the health of children, adults, and families across the nation. When messages in interventions are framed as narratives, they elicit more emotional reactions as opposed to just informationally focused messages (McQueen & Kreuter, 2010).

Perhaps one of the most long-running and successful examples, and thus an exemplar for translational scholars, is the federally funded Drug Resistance Strategies (DRS) Project led by Drs. Michael Hecht and Michelle Miller-Day since the late 1980s. Their research was initiated to understand adolescents' experiences to develop ways for them to refuse drug offers. They used narrative and performance approaches to gather the adolescents' voice to develop the *keepin' it REAL* school-based drug prevention curriculum now implemented in many states and adopted by the D.A.R.E. program. The program has been shown to have long-term effects in reducing youths' acceptance of drug use (see Hecht, Colby, & Miller-Day, 2010; Hecht & Miller-Day, 2010).

Dr. Wayne Beach's efforts in this realm will likely become an exemplar of translating research to practice in the world of oncology and family communication. His world-renowned NCI-funded cancer research (Conversations About Cancer Project [CAC]) used family phone recordings to capture how they navigated cancer (Beach & Anderson, 2003a, 2003b). The CAC research has recently been translated into *The Cancer Play*. I was incredibly moved and inspired when I had the opportunity to view a DVD screening of the play at the DC Health Communication Conference in March 2013. Dr. Beach is using the play to educate patients, family members, and medical practitioners. He and colleagues have already tested both live performances and DVDs of the play for translational efficacy; they found that after viewing, audience members' opinions were positively impacted on the importance of family communication when coping with the disease (Beach et al., 2013).

Likewise, health communication scholar, Dr. Lynn Harter, has long engaged in studies about pediatric cancer, family interaction, and provider communication from a narrative perspective. She has collaborated with oncologists at MD Anderson Cancer Center to conduct research and co-create *The Art of the Possible*, a documentary based on five families' own video footage (and, thus, a story from the family's point of view) about trying to cultivate a "a new normal" after a cancer diagnosis during childhood (for a review, see Yamasaki, 2012). I had the opportunity to view this profoundly insightful film at her narrative workshop conducted with Dr. Margaret Quinlan at the 2013 National Communication Association convention. According to Harter, the film serves to "get the conversation started" about what families face. They approached the film "as a glimpse into the narrative sense-making/memory creation process that families go through when dealing with dramatic life circumstances. It takes the film away from being a clinical look at health care and humanizes the whole endeavor."

Research that is translated into narrative form can serve a multitude of functions for breast cancer patients and their families—from allowing women to make sense of and heal from their experiences, to educating and changing opinions, to enhancing oncology care, to effecting changes in health-promotion behavior in terms of engaging in screening activities such as mammograms (Langellier & Peterson, 2004). Communication scholars have long advocated for and demonstrated the important role of narratives to our health and healing (see Harter, Japp, & Beck, 2005). The potential "healing power" of narratives is indisputable and rather has been widely documented and accepted in interventions within the medical community (Sunwolf, Frey, & Keränen, 2005).

However, to date, no research has been disseminated for the purpose of telling the breast cancer story from the mother-daughter perspective. The authentic accounts of mother-daughter coping presented in this book can be used to not only give voice to this aspect of the disease experience, but to foster healthier communication among diagnosed women and their mothers/daughters by using their stories as tools to effect behavioral modeling and advance clinical training.

In this final chapter, I advocate for taking this research a step forward and suggest ways to further translate the research into practice and enhance psycho-oncology care. While I hope to myself engage in these translational efforts, I also offer scholars and interventionists current models of translational research used in behavioral modeling and clinical training to demonstrate how these and other family narratives might be implemented into practice.

Behavioral Modeling and Narratives

Narratives are effective in communicating cancer-related information and teaching people healthy behavior. As Green (2006) states:

> Transportation into narrative worlds, or immersion into a story, is a primary mechanism of narrative persuasion. . . . [Narratives] facilitate the mental simulation of unknown, difficult, or frightening procedures (e.g., screening) and provide role models for behavior change. (p. 163)

Scholars drawing on social cognitive theory (Bandura, 1977) or transportation theories such as the transportation-imagery model (see Green & Brock, 2000) identify narratives as useful in providing models of behavior as they can inspire individuals to enact certain behaviors. According to Green (2006), "When individuals identify with characters, these characters may provide templates for 'possible selves'" (p. 167).

Narratives from this research could serve to educate and provide models to newly diagnosed mothers and daughters of healthy mother-daughter coping behavior. Excerpts from the interviews, diaries, and diary interviews can be used to create multiple stories of mother-daughter coping that are mindful of important factors that lead to variance in women's experiences, such as age or generational diversity, the cancer issue at hand, the phase of the cancer continuum, and the relational role of mother or daughter. With multiple stories, women could more easily find narratives that mirror their experiences. Additionally, by using the mother-daughter recollections in this way, families can be forewarned about issues critical to healthy coping, such as disease stressors they may encounter, their mother or daughter's communication preferences and needs (and their own), and communication dilemmas that may arise across the disease trajectory. In the end, these stories can simultaneously offer families educational insight and provide mothers and daughters the opportunity to become more aware and empathetic of each other's perspectives and needs.

At the same time, these narratives can also serve as tools in effecting behavioral change in families. For instance, Dr. Matthew Kreuter's wealth of invaluable work in breast cancer prevention has shown the power of story in getting women to engage in risk-reduction behavior such as mammogram screening (e.g., Kreuter et al., 2008). His work with African American women has shown that narrative is a particularly valuable tool in effecting behavior change for women. The stories collected and presented within this book attend to breast cancer across the life span. As such, these storied illustrations may be especially useful in teaching healthy coping behavior to mothers and daughters who encounter the disease at various developmental life phases. Kreuter and colleagues (2008) have found that women are most likely to be positively influenced by the story when they view those characters (or mothers and daughters) as "similar to themselves."

Cancer centers, hospitals, and community organizations alike may be interested in such psychosocial resources to support families. For instance, nonprofit organizations, such as Mothers Supporting Daughters with Breast Cancer (MSDBC: www.mothersdaughters.org), sometimes offer women and their families guidebooks and pamphlets, such as MSDBC's booklets for mothers and daughters on cancer resources and coping issues. Similar psychosocial interventions could be created using the narratives in this book. Implementing the storied messages into various forms may be more efficacious in teaching mothers and daughters healthy coping. For example, while guidebooks may be appealing to some women, others may prefer DVDs or videos of women portraying the mother-daughter stories of healthy coping behavior as well as unhealthy communication. Some mother-daughter pairs may prefer an interactive DVD in which they watch women telling their stories and then can discuss them together with a discussion guide or workbook document (Fisher et al., 2014), an approach that has been successfully implemented in other psycho-social, health films (e.g., see Dr. Victoria Mills' [2001] documentary *Mothers and Daughters: Mirrors That Bind* or Kathy Leichter's [2012] film on family, suicide, and mental illness, *Here One Day*).

These tools can depict what to do when adjusting to the disease, what not to do, and why. When people are given stories that represent models of behavior, their own self-efficacy increases, meaning women can begin to believe they can enact this behavior effectively (Anderson, 2000). This is important given that families describe not knowing how to be there for one another and at times engaging in unhelpful behavior. These mother-daughter stories can provide authentic depictions of healthy family behavior, thereby increasing mothers' and daughters' communication competence when coping together.

Humanizing Illness and Medical Training

Additionally, these mother-daughter narratives represent "illness stories" that are prime for educating and training medical professionals treating women and their families faced with cancer. Using narratives in this way is driven by the field of Medical Humanities, which has emerged in the last few decades as a burgeoning interdisciplinary approach to better understand illness as a socially embedded experience, thereby humanizing medical practice. By fortifying clinical practice with Humanities, more attention is given to the human condition, the nature of suffering, the relational shared experience of illness, how culture interacts with individuals' health, and how medicine is enacted within a social context (Aull, 2009). Medical Humanities unites the art and science of medicine in an effort to ensure society is better prepared to tackle the healthcare challenges of today's world. This discipline has even been implemented into medical school training (see the University of Texas Medical Branch's Institute for the Medical Humanities, which offers the nation's first PhD in medical humanities as well as dual MD/PhD degrees).

Narratives are increasingly used in medical school curricula to educate health professionals on their patients' needs and experiences thanks, in large part, to the incredible work of physician, scholar, and founder of "narrative medicine," Dr. Rita Charon. Charon, a medical doctor with a PhD in English, pioneered the first storied approach to medical training (called

Narrative Medicine) when attempting to enhance her medical students' ability to empathize with their patients. Using literature and medicine, her approach enhances provider training through the use of patient stories. She is the founder of the first graduate program in Narrative Medicine (offered at Columbia University) and her book, *Narrative Medicine: Honoring the Stories of Illness*, has changed the face of medicine on a global level.

Her work has paved the way for the federal funding of translational projects utilizing unique collaborative models merging the Humanities with traditional medicine. For instance, Dr. Forrest Lang and colleagues at Eastern Tennessee State are leading an NCI-funded collaborative effort uniting their College of Medicine and the university's Storytelling Program to create and test training modules focused on clinical training for difficult issues in oncology care, such as breaking bad news, addressing religious or spiritual issues, and interacting with family. The training modules are based on videotaped patient and clinician interviews, and the Storytelling Program also created a play, *Dispatches from the Other Kingdom*, to portray the healing implications of narratives. Additionally, health researchers Drs. Sandra Ragan, Elaine Wittenberg-Lyles, Joy Goldsmith, and Sandra Sanchez-Reilly have created well-known narrative-based approaches to clinician training in palliative and hospice care communication (see Ragan, Wittenberg-Lyles, Goldsmith, & Sanchez-Reilly, 2008; Wittenberg-Lyles, Goldsmith, Ragan, & Sanchez-Reilly, 2010). Their federally funded ACTIVE Intervention has been successful in using technology to integrate patients and their family into hospice team meetings. Additionally, their clinical end-of-life curriculum (COMFORT) is now widely implemented and critical to elevating awareness on the importance of family communication at the end of life with issues such as health literacy, decision making, and caregiving.

Likewise, the stories woven throughout this book can be used to train psychiatrists, psychologists, therapists, social workers, family counselors, genetic counselors, and other psycho-oncology practitioners working directly with diagnosed women and their families. In line with the perspective of medical family therapy, my research can give rise to the need to embed family into medical practice and heighten familial psychosocial needs in oncology care. These mother-daughter stories can be used to develop curricula key to teaching clinicians about familial communication challenges patients encounter and, at the same time, humanize a woman's journey with her family after a breast cancer diagnosis.

CLOSING

As cancer communication expert Dr. Kreps (2012) advocated, health researchers need to "go the extra mile" and translate research to practice. We need to engage in participatory community research collaborations and "to really make a difference, health communication scholarship must provide important insights into best practices for delivering health care and promoting health" (p. 8). While my research was initiated, conducted, and presented in a manner in which to more effectively build interventions to enhance mother-daughter coping, I intend to ultimately translate the research to intervention-making with my future work. Yet it is also my hope that these final suggestions inspire others to continue utilizing the knowledge in ways that argue for and augment family-centered oncology care.

While mothers and daughters can clearly be an incredibly valuable source of support and fundamental to women's (and their families') breast cancer adjustment and coping, they, too, need our support in navigating the unchartered waters of this illness. It is my hope that, at the very least, when reading these authentic, moving, and powerful breast cancer narratives of love and resilience, mothers and daughters feel more enlightened and prepared to take on the disease together and, in so doing, write their own shared mother-daughter breast cancer story.

ABOUT THE AUTHOR

Dr. Carla L. Fisher (PhD, Penn State University, 2008) is an assistant professor at George Mason University's Department of Communication and Center for Health & Risk Communication. She is a former pre-doctoral fellow with the National Institute on Aging (NIA) and received advanced post-doctoral training in health behavior theory through co-sponsored training with the National Cancer Institute (NCI), National Institutes of Health (NIH), and Office of Behavioral and Social Sciences Research (OBSSR). Prior to joining Mason, she was co-founder and coordinator of research of the Family Communication Consortium (FCC) at Arizona State University, where she remains affiliate faculty. She is also an affiliate member of Georgetown's Fisher Center for Familial Cancer Research. Using a life-span, developmental framework, she examines the adaptive functioning of family communication particularly when coping with aging and health transitions, during family-provider-patient interactions, and in terms of therapeutic and long-term physical and mental health outcomes. Her work has been funded at the federal, private, and local levels and published in research books and journals such as *Health Communication*, *Qualitative Health Research*, *Journal of Family Communication*, and the *Journal of Genetic Counseling*. She has been invited to speak internationally and nationally at cancer symposiums, health conferences, as well as medical schools and institutions about her research on mother-daughter communication, breast cancer coping, and health-promotion behavior. This research has been honored with national research awards, including the Sandra Petronio Family Communication Dissertation of the Year Award, and the National Communication Association's Communication & Aging Division's Dissertation of the Year. She continues to collaborate with leading medical institutions such as Mayo Clinic and Memorial Sloan-Kettering Cancer Center. Her mother-daughter breast cancer research website is www.motherdaughterbreastcancer.com.

REFERENCES

Afifi, T. D., Hutchinson, S., & Krouse, S. (2006). Toward a theoretical model of communal coping in postdivorce families and other naturally occurring groups. *Communication Theory, 16*, 378–409.

Afifi, T. D., & Nussbaum, J. F. (2006). Stress and adaptation theories: Families across the life span. In D. O. Braithwaite & L. A. Baxter (Eds.), *Engaging theories in family communication: Multiple perspectives* (pp. 276–292). Thousand Oaks, CA: Sage.

AHRQ. (2001). *Translating research into practice (TRIP)-II: Fact sheet.* Agency for Healthcare Research and Quality, Rockville, MD. http://www.ahrq.gov/research/findings/factsheets/translating/tripfac/index.html

Albrecht, T. L., & Goldsmith, D. J. (2003). Social support, social networks, and health. In T. L. Thompson, A. M. Dorsey, K. I. Miller, & R. Parrott (Eds.), *Handbook of health communication* (pp. 263–284). Mahwah, NJ: Lawrence Erlbaum Associates.

Anderson, B. L., Kiecolt-Glaser, J. K., & Glaser, R. (1999). A biobehavioral model of cancer stress and disease course. In R. M. Suinn & G. R. VandenBos (Eds.), *Cancer patients and their families: Readings on disease course, coping, and psychological interventions* (pp. 3–31). Washington, DC: American Psychological Association.

Anderson, R. B. (2000). Vicarious and persuasive influences on efficacy expectations and intentions to perform breast self-examination. *Public Relations Review, 26*, 97–114.

Arnett, J. J. (2000). Emerging adulthood: A theory of development from the late teens through the twenties. *American Psychologist, 55*, 469–480.

Arora, N. K., Street, R. L., Epstein, R. M., & Butow, P. N. (2009). Facilitating patient-centered cancer communication: A road map. *Patient Education and Counseling, 77*(3), 319–321.

Atlas.ti Scientific Software Development GmbH. (2010). Atlas.ti. (Version 6) [Computer software]. Berlin, Germany.

Aull, F. (2009). Medical humanities: Mission statement [Online Medical Humanities Resource hosted at the New York University School of Medicine]. Available at http://medhum.med.nyu.edu/

Baider, L. E., Cooper, C. L., & Kaplan De-Nour, A. E. (2000). *Cancer and the family* (2nd ed.). Chichester, England: Wiley.

Baider, L. E., & Kaplan De-Nour, A. (2000). Introduction. In L. Baider, G. L. Cooper, & A. Kaplan De-Nour (Eds.), *Cancer and the family* (2nd ed., pp. xxiii–xxv). Chichester, England: Wiley.

Baltes, P. B. (1987). Theoretical propositions of life-span developmental psychology: On the dynamics between growth and decline. *Developmental Psychology, 23*, 611-626,

Baltes, P. B., Reese, H. W., & Nesselroade, J. R. (1988). *Introduction to research methods: Life-span developmental psychology*. Hillsdale, NJ: Lawrence Erlbaum Associates.

Bandura, A. (1977). *Social learning theory*. Englewood Cliffs, NJ: Prentice-Hall.

Banning, J. H. (2003, July). *Ecological sentence synthesis*. Available at http://mycahs.colostate.edu/James.H.Banning/PDFs/Ecological%20Sentence%20Syntheis.pdf

Barbee, A. P., Derlega, V. J., Sherburne, S. P., & Grimshaw, A. (1998). Helpful and unhelpful forms of social support for HIV-positive individuals. In V. J. Derlega & A. P. Barbee (Eds.), *HIV and social interaction* (pp. 83–105). Thousand Oaks, CA: Sage.

Barrera, M. (1989). Models for social support and life stress: Beyond the buffering hypothesis. In L. H. Cohen (Ed.), *Life events and psychological functioning: Theoretical and methodological issues* (pp. 211–236). Newbury Park, CA: Sage.

Barrera, M. (1981). Social support in the adjustment of pregnant adolescents. In B. H. Gottlieb (Ed.), *Social networks and social support* (pp. 69–96). Beverly Hills, CA: Sage.

Barrera, M., Sandler, I. N., & Ramsay, T. B. (1983). Preliminary development of a scale of social support: Studies on college students. *American Journal of Community Psychology, 9*, 435–447.

Baxter, L. A. (2011). *Voicing relationships: A dialogic perspective*. Thousand Oaks, CA: Sage.

Baxter, L. A., Braithwaite, D. O., & Nicholson, J. H. (1999). Turning points in the development of blended families. *Journal of Social and Personal Relationships, 16*, 291–313.

Baxter, L. A., & Bullis, C. (1986). Turning points in developing romantic relationships. *Human Communication Research, 12*, 469–493.

Baxter, L. A., & Montgomery, B. M. (1996). Relating: Dialogues & dialectics. New York: Guilford Press.

Beach, W., & Anderson, J. K. (2003a). Communication and cancer? Part I: The noticeable absence of interactional research. *Journal of Psychosocial Oncology, 21*, 1–23.

Beach, W., & Anderson, J. K. (2003b). Communication and cancer? Part II: Conversation analysis. *Journal of Psychosocial Oncology, 21*, 1–22.

Beach, W. A., Buller, M. K., Dozier, D. M., Buller, D. B., & Gutzmer, K. (2013). The Conversations About Cancer (CAC) project: Assessing feasibility and audience impacts from viewing *The Cancer Play*. *Health Communication* (ahead-of-print), 1–11.

Bengston, V. L., & Harootyan, R. A. (1994). *Intergenerational linkages: Hidden connections in American society*. New York: Springer.

Berlin, K. L. (2008). *Psychological and biological stress during mother-daughter communication about breast cancer risk*. Unpublished doctoral dissertation, Vanderbilt University, Nashville, TN.

Berry, D. S., & Pennebaker, J. W. (1998). Nonverbal and verbal emotional expression and health. In G. A. Fava & H. Freyberger (Eds.), *Handbook of psychosomatic medicine* (pp. 69–83). Madison, WI: International Universities Press.

Bloom, J. R. (1982). Social support, accommodation to stress and adjustment to breast cancer. *Social Science and Medicine, 16*, 1329–1338.

Bloom, J. R., & Kessler, L. (1994). Emotional support following cancer: A test of the stigma and social activity hypotheses. *Journal of Health and Social Behavior, 35*, 118–133.

Boehmer, U., & Clark, J. A. (2001). Communication about prostate cancer between men and their wives. *The Journal of Family Practice, 50*, 226–231.

Bowlby, J. (1979). *The making and breaking of affectional bonds*. London: Tavistock.

Boyer, B. A., Bubel, D., Jacobs, S. R., Knolls, M. L. et al. (2002). Posttraumatic stress in women with breast cancer and their daughters. *The American Journal of Family Therapy, 30*, 323–338.

Braithwaite, D. O., McBride, M. C., & Schrodt, P. (2003). "Parent teams" and the everyday interactions of co-parenting in stepfamilies. *Communication Reports, 16*, 93–111.

Bronfenbrenner, U. (1979). *The ecology of human development*. Cambridge, MA: Harvard University Press.

Burles, M. C. (2006). *Mothers and daughters' experiences of breast cancer: Family roles, responsibilities, and relationships*. Unpublished doctoral dissertation, University of Saskatchewan, Saskatoon, Saskatchewan, Canada. Retrieved January 1, 2007, from http://library2.usask.ca/theses/available/etd-11222006-150720/

Burleson, B. R., Albrecht, T. L., Sarason, I. G., & Goldsmith, D. J. (1994). Introduction: The communication of social support. In B. R. Burleson, T. L. Albrecht, & I. G. Sarason (Eds.), *Communication of social support: Messages, interactions, relationships, and community* (pp. xi–xxx). Thousand Oaks, CA: Sage.

Bylund, C., Fisher, C. L., Brashers, D., Edgerson, S., Glogowski, E. A., Boyar, S. R., Kemel, Y., Siegel, B., Spencer, S., & Kissane, D. (2012). Sources of uncertainty about daughters' breast cancer risk that emerge during genetic counseling consultations. *Journal of Genetic Counseling, 12*, 292–304.

Bylund, C. L., Galvin, K. M., & Gaff, C. L. (2010). Principles of family communication. In C. Gaff & C.L. Bylund (Eds.), *Family communication about genetics* (pp. 3–17) New York: Oxford University Press.

Caplan, G. (1974). *Support systems and community mental health*. New York: Behavioral Publishing.

Carstensen, L. L. (1991). Selectivity theory: Social activity in life-span context. *Annual Review of Gerontology and Geriatrics, 11*, 195–217.

Carstensen, L. L. (1992). Social and emotional patterns in adulthood: Support for socioemotional selectivity theory. *Psychology and Aging, 7*, 331–338.

Carstensen, L. L., & Fredrickson, B. L. (1998). Socioemotional selectivity in healthy older people and younger people living with the human immunodeficiency virus: The centrality of emotion when the future is constrained. *Health Psychology, 17*, 1–10.

Carstensen, L. L., Isaacowitz, D. M., & Charles, S. T. (1999). Taking time seriously: A theory of socioemotional selectivity. *American Psychologist, 54*, 165–181.

Caughlin, J. P., & Golish, T. D. (2002). An analysis of the association between topic avoidance and dissatisfaction: Comparing perceptual and interpersonal explanations. *Communication Monographs, 69*, 275–295.

Caughlin, J. P., & Petronio, S. (2004). Privacy in families. In A. L. Vangelisti (Ed.), *Handbook of family communication* (pp. 379–412). Mahwah, NJ: Lawrence Erlbaum Associates.

Chalmers, K., Thomson, K., & Degner, L. F. (1996). Information, support, and communication needs of women with a family history of breast cancer. *Cancer Nursing, 19*, 204–213.

Charon, R. (2006). *Narrative medicine: Honoring the stories of illness*. Oxford, England: Oxford University Press.

Chernin, K. (1999). *The woman who gave birth to her mother: Tales of transformation in women's lives*. London: Penguin Books.

Cicirelli, V. G. (1983). Adult children's attachment and helping behavior to elderly parents: A path model. *Journal of Marriage and the Family, 45*, 815–822.

Cicirelli, V. G. (1991). Sibling relationships in adulthood. In S. P. Pfeifer & M. B. Sussman (Eds.), *Families: Intergenerational and generational connections* (pp. 291–310). New York: Haworth Press.

Clark, R. A., & Delia, J. G. (1979). Topoi and rhetorical competence. *The Quarterly Journal of Speech, 65*, 187–206.

Cobb, S. (1976). Social support as a moderator of life stress. *Psychosomatic Medicine, 38*, 300–314.

Cohen, M., Klein, E., Kuten, A., Fried, G., Zinder, O., & Pollack, S. (2002). Increased emotional distress in daughters of breast cancer patients is associated with decreased natural cytotoxic activity, elevated levels of stress hormones and decreased secretion of Th1 cytokines. *International Journal of Cancer, 100*, 347–354.

Cohen, M., & Pollack, S. (2005). Mothers with breast cancer and their adult daughters: The relationship between mothers' reaction to breast cancer and their daughters' emotional and neuroimmune status. *Psychosomatic Medicine, 67*, 64–71.

Compas, B. E., Worsham, N. L., Epping-Jordan, J. E., Grant, K. E., Mireault, G., Howell, D. C. et al. (1999). When mom or dad has cancer: Markers of psychological distress in cancer patients, spouses, and children. In R. M. Suinn & G.

R. VandenBos (Eds.), *Cancer patients and their families: Readings on disease course, coping, and psychological interventions* (pp. 291–308). Washington, DC: American Psychological Association.

Conrath, D. W., Higmethod, C. A., & McClean, R. J. (1983). A comparison of reliability of questionnaire versus diary data. *Social Networks, 5*, 317.

Corti, L. (1993). Using diaries in social research. *Social Research Update, 2.* Retrieved November 2, 2006, from http://www.soc.surrey.ac.uk/sru/SRU2.html

Cowan, P. A. (1991). Individual and family life transitions: A proposal for a new definition. In P. A. Cowan & E. M. Hetherington (Eds.), *Family transitions. Family Research Consortium: Advances in family research* (pp. 3–30). Hillsdale, NJ: Lawrence Erlbaum Associates.

Creswell, J. W. (2007). *Qualitative inquiry and research design.* Thousand Oaks, CA: Sage.

Creswell, J. W., & Clark, V. L. P. (2007). *Designing and conducting mixed methods research.* Thousand Oaks, CA: Sage.

Crosby, R. A., Kegler, M. C., & DiClemente, R.J. (2009). Theory in health promotion practice and research. In R. J. DiClemente, R. A. Crosby, & M. C. Kegler (Eds.), *Emerging theories in health promotion practice and research* (pp. 3-18). San Francisco, CA: John Wiley & Sons.

Dakof, G. A., & Taylor, S. E. (1990). Victim's perceptions of social support: What is helpful from whom? *Journal of Personality and Social Psychology, 58*, 80–89.

Daly, K. J. (2007). *Qualitative methods for family studies and human development.* Thousand Oaks, CA: Sage.

Daniel, C., Cieszinski, R., & Biank, N. (2007), *It's not about you: A mother and daughter's journey.* Batelier Publishing.

Datta, L. (1997). Multimethod evaluations. In E. Chelimsky & W. R. Shadish (Eds.), *Evaluation for the 21st century* (pp. 344–359). Thousand Oaks, CA: Sage.

David, H. P. (1999). Coping with cancer: A personal odyssey. In R. M. Suinn & G. R. VandenBos (Eds.), *Cancer patients and their families: Readings on disease course, coping, and psychological interventions* (pp. 373–378). Washington, DC: American Psychological Association.

Davison, K. P., & Pennebaker, J. W. (1996). Social psychosomatics. In E. T. Higgins & A. Kruglanski (Eds.), *Social psychology: Handbook of basic principles* (pp. 102–130). New York: Guilford Press.

De Raeve, L. (1997). Positive thinking and moral oppression in cancer care. *European Journal of Cancer Care, 6*, 249–256.

Dean, K. (1996). Using theory to guide policy relevant health promotion research. *Health Promotion International, 11*, 19–26.

Dedert, E., Lush, E., Chagpar, A., Dhabhar, F. S., Segerstrom, S. C., Spiegel, D., & Sephton, S. E. (2012). Stress, coping, and circadian disruption among women awaiting breast cancer surgery. *Annals of Behavioral Medicine, 44*, 10–20.

Dickson, F., & Webb, L. (Eds.). (2012). *Communication for families in crisis: Theories, research, & strategies.* New York: Peter Lang.

Donovan-Kicken, E., & Caughlin, J. P. (2010). A multiple goals perspective on topic avoidance and relationship satisfaction in the context of breast cancer. *Communication Monographs, 77*, 231–256.

Donovan-Kicken, E., & Caughlin, J. P. (2011). Breast cancer patients' topic avoidance and psychological distress: The mediating role of coping. *Journal of Health Psychology, 16*, 596–606.

Douglas, H. A., Hamilton, R. J., & Grubs, R. E. (2009). The effect of BRCA testing on family relationships: A thematic analysis of qualitative interviews. *Journal of Genetic Counseling, 18*(5), 418–435.

Duck, S. W. (2008). A past and a future for relationship research. *Journal of Social and Personal Relationships, 25*, 189–200.

Dunkel-Schetter, C. (1984). Social support and cancer: Findings based on patient interviews and their implications. *Journal of Social Issues, 40*, 77–98.

Edwards, B., & Clark, V. (2004). The psychological impact of a cancer diagnosis on families: The influence of family functioning and patients' illness characteristics on depression and anxiety. *Psycho-Oncology, 13*, 562–576.

Edwards, C. (2011). What no one knows about my mother, Elizabeth Edwards. *Glamour Magazine*. Available at http://www.glamour.com/magazine/2011/10/cate-edwards-what-no-one-knows-about-my-mother-elizabeth-edwards

Ell, K. (1996). Social networks, social support and coping with serious illness: The family connection. *Social Science & Medicine, 42*, 173–183.

Ell, K., Nishimoto, R. H., Mediansky, L., Mantell, J. E., & Hamovitch, M. B. (1992). Social relations, social support, and survival among patients with cancer. *Journal of Psychosomatic Research, 36*, 531–541.

Ellingson, L. L. (2009). *Engaging crystallization in qualitative research: An introduction*. Thousand Oaks, CA: Sage.

Erikson, E. H. (1963). *Childhood and society* (2nd ed.). New York: Norton.

Field, A. (2005). *Discovering statistics using SPSS* (2nd ed.). Thousand Oaks, CA: Sage.

Figueiredo, M. I., Fries, E., & Ingram, K. M. (2004). The role of disclosure patterns and unsupportive social interactions in the well-being of breast cancer patients. *Psycho-Oncology, 13*, 96–105.

Fingerman, K. L. (2003). *Mothers and their adult daughters: Mixed emotions, enduring bonds*. New York: Prometheus Books.

Fingerman, K. L., Nussbaum, J. F., & Birditt, K. S. (2004). Keeping all five balls in the air: Juggling family communication at midlife. In A. L. Vangelisti (Ed.), *Handbook of family communication* (pp. 135–148). Mahwah, NJ: Lawrence Erlbaum Associates.

Fischer, L. R. (1986). *Linked lives*. New York: Harper and Row.

Fischer, L. R. (1991). Between mothers and daughters. *Marriage and Family Review, 16*, 237–248.

Fisher, C. L. (2004). *Mothers' and daughters' perceptions of turning points that affected closeness in the relationship over time*. Unpublished master's thesis, Arizona State University, Tempe, AZ.

Fisher, C. L. (2005). *The mother-daughter bond over the life span: A turning point analysis*. Paper presented at the National Communication Association Convention, Family Communication Division, Boston.

Fisher, C. L. (2010). Coping with breast cancer across adulthood: Emotional support communication in the mother-daughter bond. *Journal of Applied Communication Research, 38*, 386–411.

Fisher, C. L. (2011). "Her pain was my pain": Mothers and daughters sharing the breast cancer journey. In M. Miller-Day (Ed.), *Family communication, connections, and health transitions: Going through this together* (pp. 57–76). New York: Peter Lang.

Fisher, C. L., Fowler, C., Canzona, M., & Peterson, E. (2013). *The utility of family communication patterns theory in cancer coping health interventions: Connecting mother-daughter openness with social, mental, and physical health outcomes.* Paper presented at the DC Area Health Communication conference, Fairfax, VA.

Fisher, C. L., Fowler, C., & Wolf, B. (in process). Secrets and sharing among mothers and daughters after a breast cancer diagnosis: The impact of openness and avoidance on healthy family coping.

Fisher, C. L., & Lucas, A. A. (2006). *"I don't want to talk about it!": Mother-daughter communication during developmentally related conflict over the life span.* Paper presented at the Eastern Communication Association, Interpersonal Interest Group, Philadelphia, PA.

Fisher, C. L., Maloney, E., Glogowski, E., Hurley, K., Edgerson, S., Lichtenthal, W. G., Kissane, D., & Bylund, C. (2014). Talking about familial breast cancer risk: Topics and strategies to enhance mother-daughter interactions. *Qualitative Health Research, 24,* 517-535.

Fisher, C., & Miller-Day, M. (2006). Communication over the life span: The mother-adult daughter relationship. In K. Floyd & M. T. Morman (Eds.), *Widening the family circle: New research in family communication* (pp. 3–19). Thousand Oaks, CA: Sage.

Fisher, C. L., Miller-Day, M., & Nussbaum, J. F. (2013). Healthy doses of positivity: Mothers' and daughters' use of positive communication when coping with breast cancer. In M. Pitts & T. J. Socha (Eds.), *Studies in positive communication* (pp. 98–113). New York: Peter Lang.

Fisher, C. L., & Nussbaum, J. F. (2012). "Linked lives": Mother-adult daughter communication after a breast cancer diagnosis. In F. C. Dickson & L. M. Webb (Eds.), *Communication for families in crisis: Theories, research, strategies* (pp. 179–204). New York: Peter Lang.

Fisher, C. L., & Nussbaum, J. F. (2014). Maximizing wellness in successful aging and cancer coping: The importance of family communication from a socioemotional selectivity theoretical perspective. *Journal of Family Communication.*

Fisher, C. L., Pipe, T. B., Wolf, B., & Piemonte, N. (in process). Communication strategies to facilitate healthy breast cancer coping for emerging adult daughters and their diagnosed mothers.

Fisher, C. L., Pipe, T. B., Wolf, B., Piemonte, N., & Canzona, M. (2012). *Enhancing mother-daughter coping and breast cancer prevention behavior: Challenging topics for emerging adult daughters.* Paper presented at European Association for Communication in Healthcare International conference, St. Andrews, Scotland.

Fisher, C. L., Pipe, T. B., Wolf, B., Piemonte, N., & Canzona, M. (in process). Difficult topics for emerging adult and adolescent daughters after Mom's breast cancer diagnosis.

Fisher, C. L., Wolf, B., Pipe, T. B., & Piemonte, N. (2012). *Managing difficult topics for mothers and daughters coping with breast cancer: Communication strategies to enhance emerging adult daughters' comfort*. Paper presented at the European Association for Communication in Healthcare International conference, St. Andrews, Scotland.

Fitzpatrick, M. A., & Ritchie, L. D. (1994). Communication schemata within the family: Multiple perspectives on family interaction. *Human Communication Research, 20*, 275–301.

Fredrickson, B. L., & Carstensen, L. L. (1990). Choosing social partners: How old age and anticipated endings make people more selective. *Psychology and Aging, 5*, 335–347.

Friday, N. (1977). *My mother/my self: The daughter's search for identity*. New York: Delta.

Funch, D. P., & Marshall, J. (1983). The role of stress, social support and age in survival from breast cancer. *Journal of Psychosomatic Research, 27*, 77–83.

Funch, D. P., & Mettlin, C. (1982). The role of support in relation to recovery from breast surgery. *Social Science and Medicine, 16*, 19–98.

Gabriel, S. (2010). *Eating pomegranates: A memoir of mothers, daughters, and the BRCA gene*. New York: Scribner.

Gaff, C. L., & Bylund, C. L. (2010). *Family communication about genetics: Theory and practice*. Oxford: Oxford University Press.

Gaff, C. L., Galvin, K. M., & Bylund, C. L. (2010). Facilitating family communication about genetics in practice. In C. Gaff & C. L. Bylund (Eds.), *Family communication about genetics* (pp. 243–272) New York: Oxford University Press.

Galvin, K. M., & Braithwaite, D. O. (2014). Theory and research from the communication field: Discourses that constitute and reflect families. *Journal of Family Theory & Review, 6*, 97-111.

Galvin, K. M., Bylund, C. L., & Brommel, B. J. (2004). *Family communication: Cohesion and change*. Boston: Allyn and Bacon.

Galvin, K. M., & Young, M. A. (2010). Family systems theory and genetics: Synergistic interconnections. In C. Gaff & C. L. Bylund (Eds.), *Family communication about genetics* (pp. 102–119) New York: Oxford University Press.

Geertz, C. (1973). *The interpretation of cultures*. New York: Basic Books.

Geffen, J. (2000). *The journey through cancer: An oncologist's seven-level program for healing and transforming the whole person*. New York: Crown Publishers.

Geller, G., Doksum, T., Bernhardt, B. A., & Metz, S. A. (1999). Participation in breast cancer susceptibility testing protocols: Influence of recruitment source, altruism, and family involvement on women's decisions. *Cancer Epidemiology Biomarkers & Prevention, 8*(4), 377–383.

Giarrusso, R., Du, F., & Bengtson, V.L. (2004). The intergenerational-stake phenomenon over 20 years. *Annual Review of Gerontology and Geriatrics, 24*, 55-76.

Glaser, B. G., & Strauss, A. L. (1967). *The discovery of grounded theory: Strategies for qualitative research*. New York: Aldine de Gruyter.

Goldsmith, D. J. (2004). *Communicating social support*. Cambridge, England: Cambridge University Press.

Goldsmith, D. J., Miller, L. E., & Caughlin, J. P. (2008). Openness and avoidance in couples communicating about cancer. *Communication Yearbook, 31*, 62–115.

Golish, T. D. (2000). Changes in closeness between adult children and their parents: A turning point analysis. *Communication Reports, 13*, 79–98.

Graham, E. E. (1997). Turning points and commitment in post-divorce relationships. *Communication Monographs, 64*, 350–368.

Gray, R. E., & Doan, B. D. (1990). Heroic self-healing and cancer: Clinical issues for the health professions. *Journal of Palliative Care, 6*, 32–41.

Green, L. A., & Seifert, C. M. (2005). Translation of research into practice: Why we can't "just do it." *The Journal of the American Board of Family Practice, 18*(6), 541–545.

Green, M. C. (2006). Narratives and cancer communication. *Journal of Communication, 56*, 163–183.

Green, M. C., & Brock, T. C. (2000). The role of transportation in the persuasiveness of public narratives. *Journal of Personal and Social Psychology, 79*, 701–721.

Greene, J.A. (2013). *Moral tribes: Emotion, reason and the gap between us and them*. New York: Penguin.

Gross, J. J., & Levenson, R. W. (1997). Hiding feelings: The acute effects of inhibiting negative and positive emotion. *Journal of Abnormal Psychology, 106*, 95–103.

Guba, E. G., & Lincoln, Y. S. (1981). *Effective evaluation: Improving the usefulness of evaluation results through responsive and naturalistic approaches*. San Francisco, CA: Jossey-Bass.

Guba, E. G., & Lincoln, Y. S. (1982). Epistemological and methodological bases of naturalistic inquiry. *Educational Communication and Technology Journal, 30*, 233–252.

Guba, E. G., & Lincoln, Y. S. (1989). *Fourth generation evaluation*. Newbury Park, CA: Sage.

Hagedoorn, M., Kuijer, R., Buunk, B. P., DeJong, G., Wobbes, T., & Sanderman, R. (2000). Marital satisfaction in patients with cancer: Does support from intimate partners benefit those who need it most? *Health Psychology, 19*, 274–282.

Hammersley, M. (1992). *What's wrong with ethnography?* London: Routledge.

Harter, L. M., Japp, P. M., & Beck, C. S. (Eds.). (2005). *Narratives, health, and healing: Communication theory, research, and practice*. Mahwah, NJ: Lawrence Erlbaum Associates.

Hecht, M. L., Colby, M., & Miller-Day, M. (2010). The dissemination of keepin' it REAL through DARE America: A lesson in disseminating health messages. *Health Communication, 25*, 585–586.

Hecht, M. L., & Miller-Day, M. A. (2010). "Applied" aspects of the drug resistance strategies project. *Journal of Applied Communication Research, 38*, 215–229.

Helgeson, V. S., & Cohen, S. (1999). Social support and adjustment to cancer: Reconciling descriptive, correlational, and intervention research. In R. M. Suinn & G. R. VandenBos (Eds.), *Cancer patients and their families: Readings on disease course, coping, and psychological interventions* (pp. 53–79). Washington, DC: American Psychological Association.

Hershberg, S. G. (2006). Pathways of growth in the mother-daughter relationship. *Psychoanalytic Inquiry, 26*, 56–69.

Hill, R. (1949). *Families under stress*. New York: Harper & Brothers.

Hill, R. (1958). Generic features of families under stress. *Social Casework, 31*, 139–150.

Hilton, B. A. (1994). Family communication patterns in coping with early breast cancer. *Western Journal of Nursing Research, 16*, 366–392.

Hilton, M. E. (1989). A comparison of a prospective diary and two summary recall techniques for recording alcohol consumption. *British Journal of Addiction, 84*, 1085–1092.

Horowitz, M., Wilner, N., & Alvarez, W. (1979). Impact of Event Scale: A measure of subjective stress. *Psychosomatic Medicine, 41*, 209–218.

House, J. S. (1981). *Work stress and social support*. Reading, MA: Addison-Wesley.

House, J. S., & Kahn, R. L. (1985). Measures and concepts of social support. In S. Cohen & L. Syme (Eds.), *Social support and health* (pp. 83–108). Orlando, FL: Academic Press.

Hoyert, D. L., Kung, H. C., & Smith, B. S. (2005). *National vital statistics reports: Deaths: Preliminary data for 2003*. Washington, DC: U.S. Department of Health and Human Services, National Center for Health Statistics, Center for Disease Control and Prevention, National Vital Statistics System.

Hummert, M. L., Nussbaum, J. F., & Wiemann, J. M. (1994). Interpersonal communication and older adulthood: An introduction. In M. L. Hummert, J. M. Wiemann, & J. F. Nussbaum (Eds.), *Interpersonal communication in older adulthood: Interdisciplinary theory and research* (pp. 1–14). Thousand Oaks, CA: Sage.

Huston, T. L., McHale, S. M., & Crouter, A. C. (1986). When the honeymoon's over: Changes in the marriage relationship over the first year. In R. Gilmour & S. Duck (Eds.), *The emerging field of personal relationships* (pp. 109–132). Hillsdale, NJ: Lawrence Erlbaum Associates.

Jamison, K. R., Wellisch, D. K., & Pasnau, R. O. (1978). Psychosocial aspects of mastectomy: The woman's perspective. *American Journal of Psychiatry, 135*, 434–436.

Jemel, A., Murray, T., Samuels, A., Kaplan, A. G., Miller, J. B., Stiver, I. P., & Sorrey, J. L. (2003). Cancer statistics, 2003. *CA: A Cancer Journal for Clinicians, 53*, 5–26.

Kahn, R. L., & Antonucci, T. C. (1980). Convoys over the life course: Attachment, roles, and social support. In P. B. Baltes & O. G. Brim (Eds.), *Life-span development and behavior* (pp. 254–283). New York: Academic Press.

Kaniasty, K., & Norris, F. H. (1997). Social support dynamics in adjustment to disasters. In S. W. Duck (Ed.), *Handbook of personal relationships* (pp. 595–619). Chichester, England: Wiley.

Kaufman, J. (1999). Adolescent females' perception of autonomy and control. In M. B. Nadien & F. L. Denmark (Eds.), *Females and autonomy: A life-span perspective* (pp. 43–72). Needham Heights, MA: Allyn & Bacon.

Kenen, R., Ardern-Jones, A., & Eeles, R. (2003). Living with chronic risk: Healthy women with a family history of breast/ovarian cancer. *Health, Risk & Society, 5*, 315–331.

Kershaw, T., Northouse, L., Kritpacha, C., Schafenaker, A., & Mood, D. (2004). Coping strategies and quality of life in women with advanced breast cancer and their family caregivers. *Psychology and Health, 19*, 139–155.

Klemm, P. R. (1994). Variables influencing psychosocial adjustment in lung cancer: A preliminary study. *Oncological Nursing Forum, 21*, 1059–1062.

Koerner, A. F., & Fitzpatrick, M.A (2006). Family communication patterns theory: A social cognitive approach. In D. O. Braithwaite & L. A. Baxter (Eds.),

Engaging theories in family communication: Multiple perspectives (pp. 276–292). Thousand Oaks, CA: Sage.

Koopman, C., Hermanson, K., Diamond, S., Angell, K., & Spiegel, D. (1998). Social support, life stress, pain and emotional adjustment to advanced breast cancer. *Psycho-Oncology, 7*, 101–111.

Kratzke, C., Vilchis, H., & Amatya, A. (2013). Breast cancer prevention knowledge, attitudes, and behaviors among college women and mother–daughter communication. *Journal of Community Health, 38*, 560–568.

Kreps, G. L. (2012). Translating health communication research into practice: The importance of implementing and sustaining evidence-based health communication interventions. *Atlantic Journal of Communication, 20*, 5–15.

Kreuter, M. W., Buskirk, T. D., Holmes, K., Clark, E. M., Robinson, L., Si, X., & Mathews, K. (2008). What makes cancer survivor stories work? An empirical study among African American women. *Journal of Cancer Survivorship, 2*(1), 33–44.

Kreuter, M. W., Farrell, D. W., Olevitch, L. R., and Brennan, L. K. (2000). *Tailoring health messages: Customizing communication with computer technology*. New York: Routledge.

Kreuter, M. W., Green, M. C., Capella, J. N., Slater, W. D., & Clark, E. M. (2007). Narrative communication in cancer prevention and control: A framework to guide research and applications. *Annals of Behavioral Medicine, 33*, 221–235.

Krishnasamy, M. (1996). Social support and the patient with cancer: A consideration of the literature. *Journal of Advanced Nursing, 23*, 757–762.

Kuzel, A., & Engel, J. (2001). Some pragmatic thought on evaluating qualitative health research. In J. Morse, J. Swanson, & A. Kuzel (Eds.), *The nature of qualitative evidence* (pp. 114–138). Thousand Oaks, CA: Sage.

Kvale, S. (1989). *Issues of validity in qualitative research.* Lund, Sweden: Chartwell Bratt.

Lang, F. R., & Carstensen, L. L. (1994). Close emotional relationships in late life: Further support for proactive aging in social domain. *Psychology and Aging, 9*, 315–324.

Langellier, K., & Peterson, E. (2011). *Storytelling in daily life: Performing narrative.* Philadelphia: Temple University Press.

La Sorsa, V. A., & Fodor, I. G. (1990). Adolescent daughter/midlife mother dyad: A new look at separation and self-definition. *Psychology of Women Quarterly, 14*, 593–606.

Leichter, K. (Producer & Director). (2012). *Here one day* [Documentary]. New York: Two Suns Media.

Lewis, F. M., & Deal, L. W. (1995). Balancing our lives: A study of the married couple's experience with breast cancer recurrence. *Oncology Nursing Forum, 22*, 943–953.

Lieberman, M.D. (2013). *Social: Why brains are wired to connect.* New York: Crown.

Lifshin, L. (1992). *Tangled vines: A collection of mother and daughter poems.* New York: Harcourt.

Lincoln, Y. S., & Guba, E. G. (1985). *Naturalistic inquiry.* Beverly Hills, CA: Sage.

Lyons, R. F., Mickelson, K., Sullivan, M. J. L., & Coyne, J. C. (1998). Coping as a communal process. *Journal of Social and Personal Relationships, 15*, 579–607.

MacDonald, D. J., Sarna, L., Weitzel, J. N., & Ferrell, B. (2010). Women's perceptions of the personal and family impact of genetic cancer risk assessment: Focus group findings. *Journal of Genetic Counseling, 19*, 148–160.

Maguire, K. C. (2012). *Stress and coping in families*. Cambridge: Polity Press.

Mallinger, J. B., Griggs, J. J., & Shields, C. G. (2006). Family communication and mental health after breast cancer. *European Journal of Cancer Care, 15*, 355–361.

Maloney, E., Edgerson, S., Robson, M., Brown, R., Offit, K., Bylund, C., & Kissane, D. (2012). What women with breast cancer discuss with clinicians about risk for their adolescent daughters. *Journal of Psychosocial Oncology, 30*(4), 484–502.

Manne, S. L., Dougherty, J., Veach, S., & Kless, R. (1999). Hiding worries from one's spouse: Protective buffering among cancer patients and their spouses. *Cancer Research, Therapy and Control, 8*, 175–188.

Manne, S. L., Ostroff, J. S., Norton, T. R., Fox, K., Goldstein, L., & Grana, G. (2005). Cancer related relationship communication in couples coping with early stage breast cancer. *Psycho-Oncology, 15*, 234–247.

Manne, S. L., & Schnoll, R. (2001). Measuring supportive and unsupportive responses during cancer treatment: A factor analytic assessment of the partner responses to cancer inventory. *Journal of Behavioral Medicine, 24*, 297–321.

Matarazzo, J. D. (1980). Behavioral health and behavioral medicine: Frontiers for a new health psychology. *American Psychologist, 35*, 807-817

McBride, K. (2008). *Will ever be good enough? Healing the daughters of narcissistic mothers*. New York: Free Press.

McCubbin, H. I., & Patterson, J. M. (1982). Family adaptation to crisis. In H. I. McCubbin, A. E. Cauble, & J. M. Patterson (Eds.), *Family stress, coping, and social support* (pp. 26–47). Springfield, IL: Charles C. Thomas.

McDaniel, S. H., Hepworth, J., & Doherty, W. J. (1992). *Medical family therapy: A biopsychosocial approach to families with health problems*. New York: Basic Books.

McLeod, J. M., & Chaffee, S. H. (1972). The construction of social reality. In J. Tedeschi (Ed.), *The social influence process* (pp. 50–59). Chicago: Aldine-Atherton.

McQueen, A., & Kreuter, M. W. (2010). Women's cognitive and affective reactions to breast cancer survivor stories: A structural equation analysis. *Patient Education and Counseling, 81*, S15–S21.

Meetoo, D., & Temple, B. (2003). Issues in multi-method research: Constructing self-care. *International Journal of Qualitative Methods, 2*(3). Retrieved May 30, 2007, from http://www.ualberta.ca/~iiqm/backissues/2_3final/html/meetootemple.html.

Michie, S., & Abraham, C. (2004). Interventions to change health behaviours: Evidence-based or evidence-inspired? *Psychology and Health, 19*, 29–49.

Miller-Day, M. (2004). *Communication among grandmothers, mothers, and adult daughters: A qualitative study of maternal relationships*. Mahwah, NJ: Lawrence Erlbaum Associates.

Miller-Day, M. (Ed.). (2011). *Family communication, connections, and health transitions: Going through this together*. New York: Peter Lang.

Miller-Day, M., & Fisher, C. L. (2008). Parent-emerging adult child communication and disordered eating patterns. *International Journal of Psychology Research, 3*(3), 223–248.

Miller-Day, M., Fisher, C. L., & Stube, J. (2013). Mother-daughter and son communication. In M. T. Morman & K. Floyd (Eds.), *Widening the family circle: New research in family communication* (2nd ed., pp. 1–17). Thousand Oaks, CA: Sage.

Mills, V. (Producer & Director), & Leichter, K. (Producer). (2001). *Mothers and daughters: Mirrors that bind* [Documentary]. New York: VSM Productions, LLC.

Morse, J. M. (1999). Myth #93: Reliability and validity are not relevant to qualitative inquiry. *Qualitative Health Research, 9*, 717.

Morse, J. M., Barrett, M., Mayan, M., Olson, K., & Spiers, J. (2002). Verification strategies for establishing reliability and validity in qualitative research. *International Journal of Qualitative Methods, 1(*2), Article 2. Retrieved May 23, 2007, from http://www.ualberta.ca/~ijqm/Motram, 2003.

Morse, J. M., & Niehaus, L. (2009). *Mixed method design: Principles and procedures.* Walnut Creek, CA: Left Coast Press.

Mosavel, M. (2012). Health promotion and cervical cancer in South Africa: Why adolescent daughters can teach their mothers about early detection. *Health Promotion International, 27*, 157-166.

Mosavel, M., & Genderson, M. W. (2013). From adolescent daughter to mother: Exploring message design strategies for breast and cervical cancer prevention and screening. *Journal of Cancer Education, 28*, 558-564.

Mottram, S. A. (2003). *Aging mother-adult daughter relationships solidarity, conflict, ambivalence, typology, and variations in time.* Unpublished doctoral dissertation, Middle East Technical University, Ankara, Turkey..

National Institutes of Health. (2011, August 23). NIH releases best practices for combining qualitative and quantitative research. *NIH News.* http://www.nih.gov/news/health/aug2011/od-23a.htm

Neugarten, B. L. (1968). The awareness of middle-age. In B. L. Neugarten (Ed.), *Middle age and aging* (pp. 93–98). Chicago: University of Chicago Press.

Northouse, L. (1994). Breast cancer in younger women: Effects on interpersonal and family relations. *Journal of the National Cancer Institute Monographs, 16*, 183–190.

Nussbaum, J. F. (Ed.). (1989). *Life-span communication: Normative processes.* Hillsdale, NJ: Lawrence Erlbaum Associates.

Nussbaum, J. F., & Friedrich, G. (2005). Instruction/developmental communication: Current theory, research, and future trends. *Journal of Communication, 55*, 578–593.

Nussbaum, J. F., Pecchioni, L. Baringer, D., & Kundrat, A. L. (2002). Lifespan communication. In W. B. Gudykunst (Ed.), *Communication yearbook 26* (pp. 366–389). Mahwah, NJ: Lawrence Erlbaum Associates.

Nussbaum, J. F., Pecchioni, L., Robinson, J. D., & Thompson, T. (2000). *Communication and aging* (2nd ed.). Mahwah, NJ: Lawrence Erlbaum Associates.

Nydegger, C. N. (1991). The development of paternal and filial maturity. In K. Pillemer (Ed.), *Parent child relations throughout life* (pp. 93–112). Hillsdale, NJ: Lawrence Erlbaum Associates.

O'Briend, M. L. (2011). Audience engagement with mother-daughter relationships in prime-time television of the 21st century: A qualitative analysis of interpretation, sensemaking, and perceived effects. *Mass Communications-Dissertations*. Paper 82.

Oktay, J. S. (2005). *Breast cancer: Daughters' tell their stories*. New York: Routledge.

Oktay, J. S., & Walter, C. A. (1991). *Breast cancer in the life course: Women's experiences*. New York: Springer.

Olson, D. H. (1993). Circumplex model of marital and family systems: Assessing family functioning. In F. Walsh (Ed.), *Normal family processes* (2nd ed., pp. 104–137). New York: Guilford.

Olson, D. H., Lavee, Y., & McCubbin, H. I. (1988). Types of families and family response to stress across the family cycle. In D. M. Klein & J. Adams (Eds.), *Social stress and family development* (pp. 16–43). New York: Guilford.

Owen, W. F. (1984). Interpretive themes in relational communication. *Quarterly Journal of Speech, 70*, 274–287.

Patenaude, A. F., DeMarco, T. A., Peshkin, B. N., Valdimarsdottir, H., Garber, J. E., . . . & Tercyak, K. P. (2013). Talking to children about maternal BRCA1/2 genetic test results: A qualitative study of parental perceptions and advice. *Journal of Genetic Counseling, 22*, 303-314.

Patenaude, A. F., Tung, N., Ryan, D. D., Ellisen, L. W., Hewitt, L., Schneider, K. A., Tercyak, K. P., Aldridge, J., & Garber, J. E. (2013). Young adult daughters of BRCA1/2 positive mothers: What do they know about hereditary cancer and how much do they worry. *Psycho-Oncology, 22*, 2024-2031.

Pecchioni, L. L., Wright, K., & Nussbaum, J. F. (2005). *Life-span communication*. Mahwah, NJ: Lawrence Erlbaum Associates.

Pederson, L. M., & Valanis, B. G. (1988). The effects of breast cancer on the family: A review of the literature. *Journal of Psychosocial Oncology, 6*, 95–118.

Pennebaker, J. W. (1990). *Opening up: The healing power of confiding in others*. New York: Guilford Press.

Pennebaker, J. W. (1995). Emotion, disclosure, and health: An overview. In J. W. Pennebaker (Ed.), *Emotion, disclosure, and health* (pp. 3–10). Washington, DC: American Psychological Association.

Pennebaker, J.W. (1997). Writing about emotional experiences as a therapeutic process. *Psychological Science, 8*, 162–166.

Pennebaker, J. W. (2003). Telling stories: The health benefits of disclosure. In J. M. Wilce, Jr. (Ed.), *Social and cultural lives of immune systems* (pp. 19–35). New York: Routledge.

Pennebaker, J. W. (2012). *Opening up: The healing power of expressing emotions*. New York: Guilford Press.

Peters-Golden, H. (1982). Breast cancer: Varied perceptions of social support in the illness experience. *Social Science and Medicine, 16*, 483–491.

Petronio, S. (2002). *Boundaries of privacy: Dialectics of disclosure*. Albany: SUNY Press.

Petronio, S. (2013). Brief status report on communication privacy management theory. *Journal of Family Communication, 13*, 6–14.

Pistrang, N., & Barker, C. (1992). Disclosure of concerns in breast cancer. *Psycho-Oncology, 1*, 182–192.

Pistrang, N., & Barker, C. (1998). Partners and fellow patients: Two sources of emotional support for women with breast cancer. *American Journal of Community Psychology, 26*, 439–456.

Pistrang, N., Barker, C., & Rutter, C. (1997). Social support as conversation: Analyzing breast cancer patients' interactions with their partners. *Social Science and Medicine, 45*, 773–782.

Porter, L. S., Keefe, F. J., Hurwitz, H., & Faber, M. (2005). Disclosure between patients with gastrointestinal cancer and their spouses. *Psycho-Oncology, 14*, 1030–1042.

Primomo, J., Yates, B. C., & Woods, N. F. (1990). Social support for women during chronic illness: The relationship among sources and types to adjustment. *Research in Nursing and Health, 13*, 153–161.

Ragan, S. L., Wittenberg-Lyles, E., Goldsmith, J., & Sanchez-Reilly, S. (2010). *Communication as comfort: Multiple voices in palliative care*. New York: Routledge.

Rastogi, M., & Wampler, K. S. (1999). Adult daughters' perception of the mother-daughter relationship: A cross-cultural comparison. *Family Relations, 48*, 327–336.

Ritchie, L. D., & Fitzpatrick, M. A. (1990). Family communication patterns: Measuring interpersonal perceptions of interpersonal relationships. *Communication Research, 17*, 523-544.

Rolland, J. (1994). *Families, illness, and disability: An integrative treatment model.* New York: Basic.

Rolland, J., & Williams, K. (2005). Toward a biopsychosocial model for 21st-century genetics. *Family Process, 44*(1), 3–24.

Rose, J. H. (1990). Social support and cancer: Adult patients' desire for support from family, friends, and health professionals. *American Journal of Community Psychology, 18*, 439–464.

Rosenberg, H. J., Rosenberg, S. D., Ernstoff, M. S., Wolford, G. L., Amdur, R. J., Elshamy, M., Bauer Wu, S. M., Ahles, T. A., & Pennebaker, J. W. (2002). Expressive disclosure and health outcomes in a prostate cancer population. *International Journal of Psychiatry in Medicine, 32*, 37–53.

Rowland, J. H. (1989). Developmental stage and adaptation: Adult model. In J. C. Holland & J. H. Rowland (Eds.), *Handbook of psychooncology: Psychological care of the patient with cancer* (pp. 25–43). New York: Oxford University Press.

Sallis, J. F., Owen, N., & Fisher, E. B. (2008). Ecological models of health behavior. *Health Behavior and Health Education: Theory, Research, and Practice, 4*, 465–486.

Sandelowski, M. (2000). Combining qualitative and quantitative sampling, data collection, and analysis techniques in mixed-method studies. *Research in Nursing & Health, 23*, 246–255.

Sandelowski, M., & Leeman, J. (2012). Writing usable qualitative health research findings. *Qualitative Health Research, 22*, 1404–1413.

Schroots, J. J. F., & Birren, J. E. (2001). The study of lives in progress: Approaches to research on life stories. In G. D. Rowles & N. E. Schoenberg (Eds.),

Qualitative gerontology: A contemporary perspective (2nd ed., pp. 51–65). New York: Springer.

Schwartz, G. E., & Weiss, S. M. (1978a). Yale Conference on Behavioral Medicine: A proposed definition and statement of goals. *Journal of Behavioral Medicine, 1*, 3-12.

Schwartz, G. E., & Weiss, S. M. (1978b). Behavioral medicine revisited: An amended definition. *Journal of Behavioral Medicine, 1*, 249-251.

Secunda, V. (1991). *When you and your mother can't be friends: Resolving the most complicated relationship of your life*. New York: Delta.

Secunda, V. (1992). *Women and their fathers*. New York: Delta.

Segrin, C. (2003). Age moderates the relationship between social support and psychosocial problems. *Human Communication Research, 29*, 317–342.

Segrin, C. (2006). Family interactions and well-being: Integrative perspectives. *Journal of Family Communication, 6*, 3–21.

Segrin, C., & Flora, J. (2011). *Family communication* (2nd ed.). New York: Routledge.

Sheehan, N. W., & Donorfio, L. M. (2002). Efforts to create meaning in the relationship between aging mothers and their caregiving daughters: A qualitative study of caregiving. *Journal of Aging Studies, 13*, 161–177.

Sinicrope, P. S., Patten, C. A., Clark, L. P., Brockman, T. A., Rock, E., Frost, M. H., & Cerhan, J. R. (2009). Adult daughters' reports of breast cancer risk reduction and early detection advice received from their mothers: An exploratory study. *Psycho-Oncology, 18*, 169–178.

Spira, M., & Kenemore, E. (2000). Adolescent daughters of mothers with breast cancer: Impact and implications. *Clinical Social Work Journal, 28*, 183–195.

Strauss, A., & Corbin, J. (1998). *Basics of qualitative research: Techniques and procedures for developing grounded theory*. Thousand Oaks, CA: Sage.

Suinn, R. M. (1999). *Cancer patients and their families: Readings on disease course, coping, and psychological interventions*. Washington, DC: American Psychological Association.

Suitor, J. J., & Pillemer, K. (2000). Did mom really love you best? Developmental histories, status transitions and parental favoritism in later life families. *Motivation and Emotion, 24*, 105–120.

Sunwolf, Frey, L. R., & Keränen, L. (2005). Healing effects of storytelling and storylistening in the practice of medicine. In L. M. Harter, P. M. Japp, & C. S. Beck (Eds.), *Narratives, health, and healing: Communication theory, research and practice* (pp. 237–258). Mahwah, NJ: Lawrence Erlbaum Associates.

Tannen, D. (2006). *You're wearing THAT? Understanding mothers and daughters in conversation*. New York: Random House.

Tarkan, L. (1999). *My mother's breast: Daughters face their mother's cancer*. Dallas, TX: Taylor Publishing Company.

Tercyak, K. P., Mays, D., DeMarco, T. A., Peshkin, B. N., Valdimarsdottir, H. B., Schneider, K. A., . . . & Patenaude, A. F. (2013). Decisional outcomes of maternal disclosure of BRCA1/2 genetic test results to children. *Cancer Epidemiology Biomarkers & Prevention, 22*, 1260-1266.

Tesch, R. (1990). *Qualitative research: Analysis types and software tools*. London: Falmer.

Thotis, P. A. (1985). Social support and psychological well-being: Theoretical possibilities. In I. G. Sarason & B. R. Sarason (Eds.), *Social support: Theory, research, and applications* (pp. 51–72). Dordrecht, The Netherlands: Martinus Nijhoff.

Toms, E. G., & Duff, W. (2002). "I spent 1 1/2 hours sifting through one large box…": Diaries as information behavior of the archives user: Lessons learned. *Journal of American Society for Information Science and Technology, 53*, 1232–1238.

Turk, D. C., & Kerns, R. D. (Eds.). (1985). *Health, illness, and families: A life-span perspective*. New York: Wiley-Interscience.

van Manen, M. (1990). *Researching lived experience: Human science for action sensitive pedagogy*. Albany: SUNY Press.

Vangelisti, A. L., Corbin, S. D., Lucchetti, A. E., & Sprague, R. J. (1999). Couples' concurrent cognitions: The influence of relational satisfaction on the thoughts couples have as they converse. *Human Communication Research, 25*, 370–398.

Verbrugge, L. M. (1980). Health diaries. *Medical Care, 18*, 73–95.

Walsh, F. (1996). The concept of family resilience: Crisis and challenge. *Family Process, 35*, 261–281.

Walsh, F. (2006). *Strengthening family resilience*. New York: Guilford Press.

Walters, S. D. (1992). *Lives together/worlds apart: Mothers and daughters in popular culture*. Berkeley, CA: University of California Press.

Webb, L. M., & Dickson, F. C. (2012). Effective family communication for coping with crises. In F. Dickson & L. Webb (Eds.),*Communication for families in crisis: Theories, research, & strategies* (pp. 1–26). New York: Peter Lang.

Weiss, R. S. (1974). The provisions of social relationships. In Z. Rubin (Ed.), *Doing unto others: Joining, molding, conforming, helping loving* (pp. 17–26). Englewood Cliffs, NJ: Prentice-Hall.

Wiggs, C. M. (2011). Mothers and daughters: Intertwining relationships and the lived experience of breast cancer. *Health Care for Women International, 32*, 990–1008.

Wilkinson, S., & Kitzinger, C. (2000). Thinking differently about thinking positive: A discursive approach to cancer patients' talk. *Social Science & Medicine, 50*, 797–811.

Wittenberg-Lyles, E., Goldsmith, J., Ragan, S. L., & Sanchez-Reilly, S. (2010). *Dying with comfort*. Cresskill, NJ: Hampton Press.

Wolf, B. M. (2009). Alone and together: Complicating communal coping through a dialectical analysis of family coping with breast cancer. Unpublished doctoral dissertation, University of Iowa, Iowa City, IA.

Wortman, C. B., & Lehman, D. R. (1985). Reactions to victims of life crises: Support attempts that fail. In I. G. Sarason & B. R. Sarason (Eds.), *Social support: Theory, research and applications* (pp. 463–489). Dordrecht, The Netherlands: Martinus Nijhoff.

Yamasaki, J. (2012). Creating new normals in cancer care: A review of The *Art of the Possible* [motion picture] (L. M. Harter & C. Hayward, Producers). Athens, OH: Ohio University Scripps College of Communication, 2010. *Health Communication, 27*, 219–221.

Yin, R. K. (1994). Discovering the future of the case study method in evaluation research. *Evaluation Practice, 15*, 283°290.

Yin, R. K. (2003). *Case study research: Design and methods* (3rd ed.). Thousand Oaks, CA: Sage.

Zemore, R., & Shepel, L. F. (1989). Effects of breast cancer and mastectomy on emotional support and adjustment. *Social Science and Medicine, 28*, 19–27.

Zietlow, P. H., & Sillars, A. L. (1988). Life-stage differences in communication during marital conflicts. *Journal of Social and Personal Relationships, 5*, 223–245.

Zimmerman, D. H., & Wieder, D. L. (1977). The diary: Diary-interview method. *Urban Life, 5*, 479–498.

AUTHOR INDEX

SUBJECT INDEX

CPSIA information can be obtained
at www.ICGtesting.com
Printed in the USA
FFOW02n1348010514
5181FF

9 781612 891415